Sickle Cell Disease:
a psychosocial approach

Kenny Midence
Research Psychologist, MRC Social and Community
Psychiatry Unit, Institute of Psychiatry, London

and

James Elander
Senior Research Fellow, Department of Mental Health
Sciences, St George's Hospital Medical School, London

with a Foreword by

Sally C Davies, Consultant Haematologist, Central
Middlesex NHS Trust, London

Radcliffe Medical Press · Oxford and New York

© 1994 Radcliffe Medical Press Ltd
15 Kings Meadow, Ferry Hinksey Road, Oxford OX2 0DP, UK
141 Fifth Avenue, Suite N, New York, NY 10010, USA

British Library Cataloguing in Publication Data

A catalogue record for this book is available from the British Library

ISBN 1 870905 14 8

Typeset by Acorn Bookwork, Salisbury, Wiltshire
Printed and bound in Great Britain

This book is dedicated to everyone affected by sickle cell disease.

We are grateful to the Brent Sickle Cell Centre

and the Sickle Cell Society for their support,

to Radcliffe Medical Press for their commitment to the project,

and to Sally Davies for her comments on an earlier draft.

Many thanks also to Robert West and Chris McManus

for their advice and encouragement, and to everyone

who helped us along the way.

Contents

Contents

Foreword

The haemoglobinopathies rank as one of the most important world health problems, being among the most prevalent of inherited diseases worldwide. The sickle mutation, giving rise in its homozygous or compound heterozygote state to sickle cell disease with all its varied manifestations, arose independently in at least four areas of the world. Its incidence is highest in the sub-Saharan races and the peoples who have migrated from that area. It is also found in peoples from the countries surrounding the Mediterranean – in Sicily, Greece, Turkey, and Arab countries. There are areas in India with high carrier rates and, with the opening up of Eastern Europe, it is becoming clear that there are significant numbers of patients in those countries, in particular Albania.

There is a large literature in the USA, Northern Europe, and sub-Saharan Africa respecting the natural history, clinical manifestations and often early mortality associated with sickle cell disease. This book sets out the basics in these areas in order to put the psychological and social features in their true context. Sadly, 'Studies of the psychological consequences [of sickle cell disease] have been few' (Hurtig and White, 1986). The research has been carried out predominantly in the USA and is of varying methodological quality. Remarkably little work has been undertaken in Europe in this area; the research of Midence and colleagues in North London leads the field.

Over 90% of hospital admissions in people with sickle cell disease are for the acute painful vaso-occlusive crisis, yet it remains a tragedy that, at every meeting in the UK where patients and professionals meet, the cry is for improved understanding and management of the painful crisis. Very little structured work has been done in this field and it falls to the patients themselves to explore alternative strategies against a background of disbelief from many doctors. It is imperative that improved pharmaceutical strategies should be investigated and integrated within a cohesive and holistic approach to the management of sickle. Psychology has much to offer to the management of sickle pain in terms of cognitive-behavioural approaches to its management which will surely reduce hospital admissions and intake of analgesia, as well as improve patients' psychological well-being. There is evidence that this approach can be effective in the management of other chronic diseases, so we should make every effort to incorporate it into modern management of sickle.

Sickle has the potential to influence a person's social, cognitive and emotional development as well as their physical health, with profound implications for adult functioning. The impact of the disease can be felt quite differently from person to person, but in children the feeling that they are different, overprotected, and losing time from school makes normal socialization and separation from their parents difficult. Their academic performance will be affected by all of these factors and, in up to a third, may also be diminished by sickle damage to the brain which can vary from mild cognitive loss, through a loss of IQ points, to a serious stroke. It follows that optimizing the developmental opportunities for all children with sickle necessitates an understanding of the medical situation and its interaction with the other facets within their lives, as proposed by Shute and Paton (1992). It is obvious to all doctors that family, relationships and social issues impact on the patient with sickle cell disease. There is a consensus within health psychology that family interaction needs to be taken into consideration, including the environmental and social aspects of the family. We must treat patients in the full knowledge of their role in society and recognize the importance of these interactions.

I believe that, as physicians, we have to ask ourselves why the psychological and social issues in sickle cell disease have been so ignored as compared with other chronic illnesses such as diabetes, asthma, and cancer. We need to address and resolve the issues related to race and delivery of health care and research, and how they impact on the development of services for patients in Northern Europe and the USA. I hope readers of this book will contribute to moving the field forwards.

SALLY C DAVIES
Consultant Haematologist
Central Middlesex Hospital

Introduction

Like many other chronic illnesses, sickle cell disease (SCD) has the potential for enormous disruption of normal psychosocial development, yet the psychological and social implications of the condition have received relatively little attention. Despite the fact that SCD is the most common hereditary haematological disorder, with over 5000 sufferers in the UK alone, its public profile in terms of scientific research, support services, and general public awareness is low compared with illnesses like asthma, cystic fibrosis, diabetes, and haemophilia. One of the reasons for this is probably that SCD is mainly limited to people of African, Afro-Caribbean, Mediterranean, and Middle Eastern origins. The link between SCD and ethnicity adds a political dimension to the issues raised by the condition, and compounds the feelings of isolation and lack of support that are often experienced by sufferers and their families.

This situation is slowly changing, however, and SCD is beginning to receive some of the attention and resources it should command. The World Health Organization has recognized SCD as a high priority and a major health problem. As in many other chronic illnesses, the prospects of an imminent and decisive medical breakthrough appear slim, and important targets for research and service provision are the psychological and social implications of the illness. These include the effects of SCD on the lives of sufferers, the ways in which they can adapt and learn to cope with the difficulties it imposes, and the most effective ways in which support services can be provided. Chronic illnesses present sets of difficulties and complications for those affected, many of which arise from particular characteristics of the condition. In SCD these include recurrent episodes of acute pain; limitations to activities and lifestyle; and the risk of a range of secondary medical complications, many of which are potentially fatal.

This book is a basic text on the psychological and social implications of SCD. Based on a comprehensive review of research findings in this area, it provides an analysis of how a number of major problems may affect sufferers and their families, and considers how our knowledge to date could best be implemented in preventive and supportive interventions of different kinds. The material is presented in the light of medical aspects of the condition and the experiences of sufferers and their families, with relevant comparisons with other chronic illnesses where possible.

In Chapter 1 we set out the established medical, historical, and geographical facts about the condition, which form the context of the social and psychological material presented in later chapters. These include the biological basis and inheritance of different forms of SCD; physiological aspects of the most important medical complications; prevalence and distribution of SCD worldwide; and a brief review of historical developments in our understanding of the condition.

Chapter 2 deals with research issues relevant to the investigation of psychosocial aspects of a chronic illness such as SCD. This chapter is intended to serve two purposes. The first is as a tutorial on the design and execution of such studies for workers in the field who are themselves involved, or who may wish to become involved, in conducting research in this area. The second is to alert the reader to considerations that should be taken into account when interpreting and evaluating the findings of such studies. The issues covered include the advantages and limitations of different research designs; the selection of appropriate samples and control groups; the measurement of psychological characteristics; and the interpretation of findings that indicate multiple and complex relationships among variables.

Recurrent episodes of acute pain are the principal way in which SCD manifests itself in the day-to-day lives of those affected by the condition, and Chapter 3 deals with all aspects of pain crises in SCD. These include the assessment and management of pain; the incidence and severity of pain crises in SCD; and behavioural and pharmacological methods for the prevention and management of SCD pain.

Chapter 4 considers the effects of SCD in early life among those affected. Sickle cell disease can have its most dramatic effects in childhood and adolescence, and much of the research that has been conducted on SCD has focused on young people affected by the condition. In this chapter we look at the evidence for an increased risk of problems in the areas of emotional, behavioural, and intellectual adjustment associated with SCD, and examine factors that appear to influence the extent to which young people with SCD are adversely affected. These include aspects of the disease and of the personality and family functioning of affected young people. Detailed accounts of descriptive, comparative, and correlational studies of children and adolescents with SCD are provided. We also consider the effects of SCD on the schooling and educational achievement among those affected.

Sickle cell disease can have an enormous impact on family life, and Chapter 5 examines the effects that SCD can have on the families of those affected and the roles that family members can play in the management of SCD. Topics covered include the psychological implications for the parents and siblings of affected children; the impact of SCD on family functioning and cohesiveness; the financial burden imposed on affected families by the condition; the different forms of support available to families; and the ways in which family members and overall patterns of family interaction can assist or obstruct affected individuals in their efforts to cope with SCD.

Chapter 6 focuses on the implications of SCD in adult life. This is an area that has been neglected by much of the literature on the condition, although various important aspects of adult life can be significantly affected by SCD. These include mental health and psychological adjustment; decisions to be made by carriers and sufferers about having children; choices about employment and problems in the workplace; and coping with the various medical complications of the condition that arise later in life.

The roles played by various medical and non-medical services in the support of sufferers and their families are considered in Chapter 7, with particular reference to likely or desirable changes in the way that such services will be organized and delivered in future. Such services include hospitals, Sickle Cell Centres, Social Services Departments, and formal and informal systems of support in the community. The development of more effective therapeutic interventions for SCD, such as bone marrow transplant, gene therapy, and better pain management, are considered and problems in the provision of services for SCD, including the need for attitude change amongst professionals, allocation of resources, and the need to tailor services to meet the needs of those ethnic groups most affected by SCD are examined.

Chapter 8 draws together and evaluates the material presented throughout the book and considers the findings in a wider perspective. In this chapter we review the current state of psychosocial research on SCD; consider worthwhile areas for future studies; make recommendations about service provision; and point to likely future developments in the field.

The book is aimed primarily at psychologists, social workers, counsellors, medical doctors, nurses, and other health care workers who deal with SCD in their training and practice. It should also be a relevant resource for students of health psychology and chronic illness more generally. Throughout the book we have attempted to present material in the most straightforward way possible, so that the information and analysis we offer should also be accessible to a wider readership, including those people directly affected by sickle cell disease.

1

What is Sickle Cell Disease?

Sickle cell disease (SCD) is a family of blood disorders including sickle cell anaemia (SS), SC disease (SC — a milder form), and sickle β Thalassaemia (SβThal), which have in common a tendency for red blood cells to 'sickle' – distort into a crescent shape – under certain conditions. Sickling is caused by an alteration of the haemoglobin molecules, which causes them to link up, forming stiff rods that distort the shape of the red blood cells and reduce their normal elasticity. The deformed cells can create blockages in small blood vessels (*see* Figure 1), leading to oxygen deprivation and tissue damage. All of the medical symptoms associated with sickle cell disease appear to stem from the disruption to normal circulation caused by sickled red blood cells. Effects are variable, but include chronic anaemia, recurrent attacks of pain, frequent bacterial infections, gradual deterioration of tissue and organ function, and the risk of a shortened life expectancy.

The type of haemoglobin in a person's red blood cells is determined by their genes. Sickle cell anaemia (SS) is produced when β^{S*} genes have been inherited from both parents. If a β^S gene is inherited from only one parent, and the other parent contributes the normal β^{A*} gene, the individual would have sickle cell trait (AS), and could pass on to their children either the β^S or β^A gene.

Genetic engineering or gene therapy may in future make it possible to alter an individual's genetic make up, but for the present there is no way of changing the genes that determine a person's physical characteristics. As there are at present no clinically effective methods to prevent the sickling process, medical treatment for sickle cell disease is predominantly symptomatic and supportive, consisting of alleviating pain and combatting symptoms as they occur.

---

*β^S and β^A refer to the genetic information which codes for the beta chain of the haemoglobin molecule (*see* page 10).

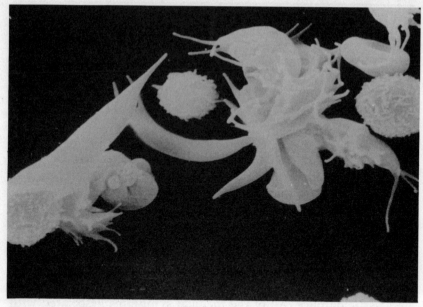

Figure 1: Sickled cells in a blood vessel (courtesy of Dr David Bevan, Department of Haematology, St George's Hospital, London).

The History of Sickle Cell Disease

The first recorded description of sickle cell disease in Africa is attributed to Africanus Horton, who in 1874 described fevers of crises, shifting joint pains, and abnormality of the blood. Before this time the illness must have been recognised for generations in West Africa. Konotey-Ahulu (1968) has described how some elderly men in Ghana could trace back relatives who had probably died of the disease over several generations. 'Cold season rheumatism' was given repetitive, onomatopoeic names such as 'Chwe-cheechwa', 'Ahututuo', 'Nuidudui', and 'Nwiiwii' by the tribes of Ghana.

Other reports in North America also described features highly suggestive of sickle cell disease. Lebby (1846) and Hodenpyl (1898) both reported autopsies in which no spleen could be found, these were conducted on a runaway slave executed for murder, and a 32-year-old man who died in hospital after complaining of pains all over the body, pleuritic symptoms, and jaundice.

The first generally accepted case report of sickle cell disease in North America took place in 1910, when Dr James Herrick of Chicago published a paper in the *Archives of Internal Medicine* entitled *Peculiar elongated and sickle-shaped red blood corpuscles in a case of severe anaemia*. He described a young student from Grenada who was studying in Chicago, and who complained of coughing and fever. Herrick examined the student's red blood cells and found the characteristic pathognomonic elongated shape, which has become identified with sickle cell disease. Other case reports followed and, in a summary of the first four, Mason (1922) coined the term 'sickle cell anaemia', concluding that this was a new disease entity.

The clinical features associated with SCD have been gradually noted by a succession of workers since the time of the first reports, and some of the personalities involved have been described by Conley (1980). In 1949, Linus Pauling identified haemoglobin S (HbS) as a molecular abnormality. This made SCD the first genetic disorder in which the molecular abnormality was precisely identified. In 1964, Makio Murayama developed a molecular hypothesis for the sickling of SS red blood cells. He suggested that, when deoxygenated, HbS molecules polymerise by means of hydrophobic interaction to form microfilaments that cause distortion of the red blood cell. This insight allowed specific tests for the presence of HbS to be devised, and opened the door for screening, counselling, and later prenatal diagnosis.

The first Sickle Cell Centre in Britain was opened in Brent, North-West London, in October 1979. The Centre has been a model for other sickle cell centres, which have been set up in other parts of the UK. The Sickle Cell Society was formed in Britain as a registered charity (also in 1979), to work directly for the relief of people suffering from SCD, and to campaign for improvements in the services available to them.

Prevalence and Distribution of Sickle Cell Disease

Sickle cell disease is the most common known hereditary blood disorder. It has been estimated that around 50 000 people suffer from sickle cell anaemia in the USA, and one baby in every 500 born in that country has the condition (Barnhart, Henry, and

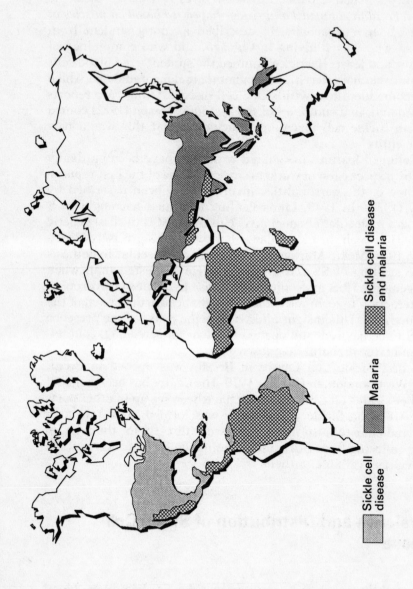

Sickle cell disease
and malaria

Malaria

Sickle cell
disease

Figure 2: Parts of the world in which SCD and malaria are most common.

Lusher, 1976). This rate rises to one in 300 babies of Afro-Caribbean origin, and one in every 60 in many African communities (Serjeant, 1992).

In Britain, people with SCD are predominantly Afro-Caribbean and West African in origin, but some are also from the Mediterranean, Middle East, and Asia. There are an estimated 4000 to 5000 people suffering from SCD in Britain (Brozovic and Davies, 1987), with around 2000 in London (Brozovic and Anionwu, 1984). Affected babies can be diagnosed at birth, and at least 150 babies with SCD are thought to be born in Britain every year (Brozovic and Davies, 1987).

Sickle cell *trait* offers some protection against malaria, so that in areas where malaria is, or was, endemic, the HbS gene can be an advantage, particularly in the very young. The reasons for this are not yet fully understood, although it is also true of other major genes for abnormal haemoglobins and for some other conditions. In the case of SCD, one possibility is that malarial parasites are unable to fully exploit sickle haemoglobin. Another is that sickling destroys red cells containing parasites. Selection for the sickle trait is also assisted by the fact that spontaneous abortion and premature birth are more frequent among women with malarial infection, and therefore less common among those with sickle cell trait (Serjeant, 1983).

Sickle cell anaemia (SS) is no protection against malaria however. Indeed, malaria is a dangerous complication for a person with sickle cell disease. Figure 2 shows the incidence of SCD worldwide, compared with the incidence of malaria. The areas most affected by SCD are Africa, North America, and the Caribbean, whereas thalassaemia is most common in the Mediterranean and the Middle East.

The Biology of Sickle Cell Disease

Sickle Haemoglobin (HbS)

Human blood consists of four elements. These are plasma, the fluid that transports the proteins and cells; white blood cells, which combat infections; platelets, which cause clotting when the circulation is breached; and red blood cells, which transport oxygen around the body. Red blood cells consist of an outer membrane containing molecules of haemoglobin. Usually the membrane is smooth and the cells are flexible. This plasticity is essential for normal blood flow in the narrow vessels of the microcirculation. The reason for the unusual features of red blood cells in people with SCD is an abnormal form of haemoglobin, called haemoglobin S (HbS).

Haemoglobin is a molecule that transports oxygen, picking it up as blood passes through the lungs and releasing it as the blood flows through the body. Normal adult haemoglobin (HbA) makes up over 95 per cent of the haemoglobin in most people over 1 year of age. The molecule has two components: (1) a pigment (heme); and (2) two protein chains (globin). These globin polypeptide chains (α and β) have a total of 574 amino acids per molecule. The exact sequence of amino acids for each chain is known, and the difference between HbA and HbS is at the number 6 position in the β chain, where valine is substituted for a glutamic acid.

There are more than a hundred other known abnormal forms of haemoglobin, and most are also the result of a single amino acid substitution in the β chain. HbS is important among these abnormal forms in that it is associated with significant clinical effects. The reason for this is that the substitution at position number 6 takes place at the external surface of the molecule, where the valine molecule can bond to leucine and phenylalanine groups on neighbouring haemoglobin molecules when oxygen is released.

Under conditions of low oxygen tension, HbS molecules tend to polymerize, or 'stack', which converts the haemoglobin from a fluid, or 'sol' state to a viscous or 'gel' state. Stiff rods of HbS are formed, leading to the deformation of red cells into an elongated or sickle shape. Polymerization will only take place, however, if a cell contains predominantly HbS molecules. Dilution of HbS with normal HbA makes the red blood cells fairly resistant to sickling, because polymerization is a result of reactions between HbS molecules. An HbS and an HbA molecule do not 'bond' in the same way as two HbS molecules. The red blood cells of a person with sickle cell anaemia (SS) generally contain between 80 and 100 per cent HbS. In people with sickle cell trait (AS) the proportion of HbS is between 45 and 55 per cent, which is generally too low to cause sickling. However, sickling can occur under certain extreme conditions in people with sickle cell trait.

HbS has several other unusual properties, which allow it to be detected in a very precise way. Its solubility is different from HbA in such a way that it can be detected by inexpensive screening tests. The many different variants of haemoglobin, including HbS,

have different electrical properties, allowing separation and identification.

Genes and Haemoglobin

Genes are chemical codes that we inherit from our parents. The
codes specify sequences of amino acids chains for the production
of complex molecules. Haemoglobin is such a molecule, and HbS
is one of several abnormal haemoglobin types resulting from
slightly different genetic coding. Others include HbC, HbD, and
HbO. As we have noted, HbS is caused by a single substitution of
one amino acid for another at one point in the chain. HbC is caused
by a different substitution (lysine) at the same point in the amino
acid chain.

Genes are arranged in pairs at particular positions (alleles)
along pairs of chromosomes. The nuclei of all somatic cells in our
bodies contain 23 pairs of chromosomes. When cells divide for the
purpose of regeneration and growth (mitosis), the two chromosomes in each pair separate and each replicates the missing half,
so that two versions of the original are formed. Cell division for
the purpose of creating germ cells (the ovum in the female and
spermatozoa in the male) is a slightly different process called
meiosis. Here, pairs of chromosomes separate but do not replicate,
so that each new germ cell contains only half of the full package
of genetic information needed to make a new individual. At conception the two halves combine and the genetic make up of the
new person is sealed, including whether they will suffer from, or
carry, a form of sickle cell disease.

Genes generally function in either a 'dominant' or 'recessive'
manner. When a dominant gene is paired with a recessive gene (a
'heterozygous' condition), the dominant gene is 'expressed' to a far
greater extent. For a recessive gene to be fully expressed, it must
be paired with a similar recessive gene (a 'homozygous' condition).
This affects the extent to which information contained in our genes
is expressed in our physiology. The gene for HbA is dominant,
whereas those for HbS and HbC are recessive, which is the reason
why the full form of sickle cell disease must be inherited from both
parents. If it is inherited from only one parent, and the other
parent contributes genes for normal haemoglobin (HbA), the gene
for sickle haemoglobin will be partially expressed, but clinical
symptoms do not occur as most of the haemoglobin in the red
blood cells of the child will reflect the (dominant) normal coding

for HbA. The gene coding for HbS can, however, be passed on to that person's own children, where it would lead to sickle cell anaemia if it were then combined with another gene for HbS.

Haemoglobin Variants

Because genes are inherited from both parents, codes for different forms of haemoglobin can be combined in any one individual with those that code for HbA and HbS. Some of the most important combinations are the normal AA, AC trait, SC disease, CC disease, sickle cell trait (AS), homozygous SS or sickle cell anaemia, and SβThalassaemia. AA is normal healthy haemoglobin, in which the genes for HbA have been inherited from both parents. Combinations of HbS and other variants, or βThalassaemia, are responsible for the range of the severe forms of SCD.

Sickle Cell Trait
AS is sickle cell trait, in which individuals are well and without symptoms except under extreme conditions. They carry the HbS gene throughout their lives and can pass it on to their children. Depending upon the gene inherited from the second parent, their children risk either becoming carriers themselves, or suffering the full (SS) or another (e.g. SC) form of SCD. Eight to ten per cent of black Americans have been estimated to have sickle cell trait, and in parts of West Africa the incidence may be as high as 45 per cent. It is in trait form that sickle haemoglobin protects against malaria.

Sickle Cell Anaemia
SS is the homozygous form of SCD, usually called sickle cell anaemia. Sufferers have inherited the genes for sickle haemoglobin (HbS) from both parents, who are either sufferers of SCD, or carriers of the trait.

Sickle β Thalassaemia
SβThalassaemia results from the gene for sickle haemoglobin (HbS) being inherited from one parent and that for β thalassaemia from the other. The clinical presentation of SβThalassaemia ranges from a very mild form of SCD to that found in sickle cell anaemia.

12

Haemoglobin C Trait
AC is haemoglobin C trait, in which the genes for normal haemoglobin have been inherited from one parent, and those for HbC from the other. People with this inheritance are asymptomatic, but can of course pass the HbC gene on to their children. It has been estimated that around 2 per cent of black Americans possess just one gene for C haemoglobin, although the highest rates have been observed in parts of West Africa.

Haemoglobin C Disease
The CC pattern of inheritance, in which both parents have passed on the genes for HbC, leads to haemoglobin C disease. The disease is uncommon, affecting an estimated one in 6000 black Americans, and gives few clinical problems. Most patients are free of symptoms, although there is sometimes a mild anaemia. Growth, development, and life expectancy are normal, although many patients have a moderately enlarged spleen and some are said to suffer from recurrent episodes of arthralgia and/or abdominal pain.

SC Disease
SC indicates that the gene for sickle haemoglobin has been combined with that for haemoglobin C. SC disease is about one-third as common as sickle cell anaemia in the UK, and affects around one person in 1500 among black Americans. Again, the incidence is higher in parts of West Africa. The clinical manifestations are very variable and generally similar to, but less severe than, sickle cell anaemia. Onset of symptoms is generally later in life, with about half of affected individuals remaining symptom-free until at least 10 years of age.

Probabilities of Inheritance

Given that an individual may possess two different β chain genes, and that the haemoglobin type inherited by any individual depends upon contributions from both parents, there is usually an element of chance in the inheritance of SCD. If both parents have sickle cell trait (AS), they can each produce germ cells containing genes either for HbA or HbS. In order for their child to inherit SS, conception would need to involve both an egg and a sperm that contained the genes for HbS. There is a one in four chance (25 per cent) of this happening, and the same odds for a conception involving both sperm and egg carrying genes for normal haemoglobin (HbA). For the child to inherit sickle cell trait however, only one gene of the type HbS would need to be involved, and the odds of this happening are one in two, or 50 per cent.

If one parent is a carrier (AS) and the other has SS, then the odds of morbidity in their children are raised to 50 per cent for inheriting SS, while 50 per cent will inherit, AS the trait form, with no possibility of their offspring being entirely free of HbS.

Where one parent is a carrier (AS) and one is free of sickle cell (AA) the odds of inheritance in their children are reversed, to 50 per cent for inheriting the trait form and 50 per cent for being free of HbS. From this pattern of parenthood a child could not be conceived that would suffer from SCD.

However, where one parent has SS and the other is free of the condition, all of their children would definitely inherit the (heterozygous) trait norm, and where both parents had SS haemoglobin, each of their offspring would be also HbSS.

The same probabilities apply for inheritance of HbC and other abnormal forms of haemoglobin, the genes for which can be inherited in combination with those for normal haemoglobin, sickle haemoglobin, or βThalassaemia.

Sickle Cell Trait

Sickle cell trait is the name given to the condition in which an individual has inherited the sickle cell gene from only one parent. There is sometimes confusion about the significance of sickle cell trait (AS). AS trait is not included as a disease in the haemoglobinopathies, and it is not an illness. Sickle cell trait does not require any treatment and healthy carriers will not develop related medical problems as they get older. The trait seems to provide some protection against malaria, which is why the β^s gene has not disappeared under selective pressure, and which accounts for the geographical distribution of sickle haemoglobin.

In such individuals sickle haemoglobin (HbS) makes up only about 50 per cent of haemoglobin, which is not enough to cause anaemia or other symptoms under normal conditions, and life expectancy is generally normal. Sickling, with the effects noted for SS, can occur, but only under extreme conditions, or when several risk factors act in combination to lower oxygen tension sufficiently. Medical complications are therefore rare, but the potential risk should not be overlooked. For example, hypoventilation during general anaesthesia is dangerous, and the trait has been identified as placing military recruits at higher risk of sudden, unexplained death following physical exercise (Kark *et al.*, 1987). Splenic infarction has been reported in people with sickle cell trait when flying at high altitude in unpressurised aircraft, or after vigorous exercise at high altitude.

Any individual carrying the sickle cell trait should be aware of the risk of passing the β^s gene to their offspring. Depending on the genetic make up of the second parent, the children of a person with sickle cell trait would be at risk of carrying the trait themselves, or of inheriting the homozygous form SS.

Sickle Cell Disease as a Medical Condition

Sickle Cell Anaemia

For individuals who have inherited the 'homozygous' (SS) form of SCD, also known as sickle cell anaemia, the clinical picture is highly variable. Some children have very few pain crises and are relatively symptom-free, whereas others may require frequent hospital admissions and have a very disrupted lifestyle. In general, SCD patients live with intermittent pain that may require hospital admission for control, and are under the threat of an early and sudden death related to the disease. Symptoms of SCD can start as early as 3 to 18 months of age, and the highest death rate occurs within the first 3 years of life. Recent improvements in medical care have raised the life expectancy of people with SCD, and some patients have been reported to survive into their 50s, 60s, and 70s (Brozovic and Davies, 1987).

For the first few months of life human red blood cells are made up of between 50 and 95 per cent fetal haemoglobin (HbF), which does not sickle and interferes with gel formation by HbS molecules; initially this protects people who can go on to develop symptoms. By 6 to 12 months of age the red blood cells will be made up predominantly of haemoglobin S, and the potential for developing medical problems begins.

Infection

Sickle cell anaemia is often first detected in a young child because of a bacterial infection. Acute pneumococcal infections such as septicaemia, meningitis, pneumonia, and peritonitis are among the most common causes of death in the first 3 years of life. The risk of bacterial pneumonia is 100 times higher than normal for children with sickle cell disease, and this is the most common infection leading to hospitalization. There is also a 300-fold increase in the risk of bacterial meningitis and a 25-fold increase in risk of salmonella osteomyelitis. Increased susceptibility to infections in SCD has long been recognised, but the reasons for it are multifactorial and not completely understood at present. The spleen is an important defence against infection, and splenic function is impaired by SCD *per se*. This is because the spleen environment is viscous, hypoxaemic, and acidotic, all of which promote sickling. With repeated sickling the spleen becomes scarred, loses immunological function and eventually atrophies. 'Functional asplenia', where the circulation bypasses elements of the spleen, contributes to the increased risk of overwhelming infection.

Splenic sequestration

Splenic sequestration is common in young children but is rarely seen after the age of 5 or 6 years because of splenic atrophy. All sequestration syndromes are potentially life-threatening. Parents can be taught to palpate and examine for an enlarging spleen, to ensure prompt diagnosis and therapy (Vichinsky, 1991). An enlarged spleen observed after 7 or 8 years of age generally indicates chronic malaria, SC disease or βThalassaemia rather than sickle cell anaemia (SS).

Acute splenic sequestration is one of the most dangerous and least understood complications of SCD, and is one of the most common causes of very early death. It occurs when there is a sudden pooling of red cells into the spleen, leading to enlargement of the spleen, severe abdominal pain, acute anaemia, peripheral circulatory failure, shock, and sometimes death. The patient becomes very pale without evidence of external bleeding or infection. Treatment consists of urgent blood transfusion, intensive resuscitation, and intravenous antibiotics. Removal of the spleen should be considered as further occurrences are common (Franklin, 1990).

The central nervous system

Restricted circulation due to sickling ('vaso-occlusion') can affect almost any organ of the body. When the central nervous system (CNS) is affected, the result is a medical emergency, because even a short period of occlusion of a blood vessel in the brain can cause permanent weakness, aphasia (language impairment), convulsive disorder (epilepsy), or even death, depending upon the part of the brain affected. Urgent symptomatic treatment must be given, including intravenous fluids and exchange blood transfusions, and anticonvulsive medication (e.g. diazepam or phenobarbital) as required. Special rehabilitation treatment such as physiotherapy, speech therapy, or occupational therapy may be needed later because of permanent damage to brain tissue. Cerebrovascular accidents are found in about 7 per cent of children with SS. Most children make an excellent recovery, but unless they are offered hypertransfusion therapy over a period of years (Crawford, 1991), there is a two-thirds risk of recurrence within 36 months (Powars, 1975). The retina of the eye is made up of nerve tissue and is particularly susceptible to the effects of sickling, so that a variety of ophthalmological abnormalities can occur in patients with SCD, including decreased visual acuity and blindness.

Pain

The most common symptom of SCD is the vaso-occlusive crisis, commonly known as a pain crisis. This is the most urgent and alarming symptom of the condition from the patient's point of view. Pain crises are often preceded by infection, dehydration, acidosis, cold exposure, physical exertion, stress, or emotional disturbance, but in many cases there is no apparent precipitating event. Crises are variable in intensity, frequency, and duration but the pain, often described as 'throbbing' and accompanied by low grade fever, can be excruciating, requiring hospitalization and narcotic pain relief.

Sickle cell anaemia also causes impairment of renal concentration, so that most patients pass large quantities of urine and need to compensate by taking plenty of fluids to maintain hydration. Oral or intravenous fluids are an important part of pain crisis management, because at that time the patient is usually in a state of negative fluid balance, and dehydration promotes sickling.

Dactylitis (pain, soft tissue swelling, heat, and tenderness in the

17

hands and feet), is another way in which the condition may first present itself in young children. This has been observed from the age of 4 months with a peak incidence at 2 years of age. Other early symptoms are sometimes misdiagnosed. Joint pain, swelling, and limitation of movement occur frequently in young children and can mimic rheumatic fever, whilst abdominal pain crises, which are also common in childhood, can give the appearance of appendicitis. Very early pain crises are often put down to colic or irritability.

Bones

Vaso-occlusion caused by sickling can also affect bone tissue and skeletal development, with damage at some sites more common than at others. Dactylitis is common in young children whereas in adults the head of the femur and the humerus are more vulnerable, because the blood vessels supplying them are long and tortuous and the collateral circulation is poor. The bone marrow cavity is expanded and there may also be changes to the skull, long bones, and spine, with osteoporosis of the vertebrae in adolescents and young adults.

Anaemia

The average lifespan of an SS red blood cell is 6 to 10 days, compared with 120 in normal red blood cells. The bone marrow works to compensate for this, which allows a relatively stable haemoglobin level to be maintained, but is not sufficient to prevent chronic anaemia.

Other effects

Other medical problems frequently associated with SCD include leg ulcers and priapism (persistent painful erections). Management of leg ulcers generally consists of rest, local measures to combat infection, and, occasionally, transfusions of blood or even skin grafts. Priapism is usually treated with relaxants, pain killers, and exchange transfusions. Surgical drainage and definitive operation are sometimes used to reinstate normal circulation. These involve a risk of impotence. Priapism can clearly have disturbing psychosexual, as well as medical, implications for the sufferer (see Chapter 6).

Sickle cell disease can complicate and limits the lives of those affected by it in many different ways. This book is about the social and psychological implications of the disease, but the condition also creates problems for what would otherwise be more routine medical procedures. Certain precautions must be followed, for example, before operating surgically on a patient with SCD. Hypoxia and acidosis must be prevented, and transfusions of blood may be needed to avoid sickling crises during the operation. Anaesthetics must be used with more caution than usual. There is also a higher risk of postoperative infection.

Women with SCD suffer from delayed onset of menarche and reduced fertility. Pregnancy is another example of an otherwise routine situation that can be complicated in a woman with SCD. Early pregnancy generally does not alter the frequency and severity of crises for a woman with SCD, but problems often arise in the later stages, and the risks of premature birth, spontaneous abortion, stillbirth, and neonatal death are all reported to be increased significantly. Some patients require blood transfusions during pregnancy. Family planning must be approached sensitively and carefully because of the inherited nature of the condition, and counselling on the advisability of pregnancy and the problems it may raise is an important part of the management of the disease and support for the patient. Women with SCD have yet another factor to take into account when considering whether or not to terminate a pregnancy, and the condition also affects their choice of contraceptive (see Chapter 6).

Thalassaemia

The thalassaemia syndromes are a related group of genetically determined conditions that affect the production of normal haemoglobin chains. The genetics and biochemistry that give rise to the thalassaemias are more complex and variable than those involved in SCD. αThalassaemia (in which insuffient α chains of haemoglobin are produced) is most prevalent in parts of Asia, whereas βThalassaemia (where β chain production is reduced) is most common in parts of Sardinia, Cyprus, and around the Mediterranean, although both forms are found to some extent all around the world. Both types can exist in illness form (where the trait is inherited from both parents), in trait form (inherited from only one parent), and in combination with sickle cell.

In the latter case, the result is a moderately severe anaemia and a clinical prognosis similar to that of SS. Vaso-occlusive episodes can occur as frequently as in SS, but enlargement of the spleen is often pronounced and may persist throughout life.

SC Disease

In SC disease the gene for HbS has been combined with that for HbC. The clinical manifestations are very variable and generally similar to but less severe than in sickle cell anaemia. Onset of symptoms is generally later in life, with about half of affected individuals remaining symptom-free until about 10 years of age.

Sickle Cell Disease as a Chronic Illness

A chronic illness is one that persists over a long period and for which there is no decisive medical treatment. Treatment aims instead to reduce the effects of the disease as far as possible and enable the individual to adopt a normal life-style. Some 10 to 12 per cent of children suffer from one chronic illness or another, including asthma (the most common), congenital heart disease, chronic kidney disease, diabetes, haemophilia (another inherited blood disorder), epilepsy, rheumatoid arthritis, muscular dystrophy, and SCD. Some cause progressive deterioration whereas others (including SCD) are associated with intermittent periods of relapse and illness. Either way, patients and their families must cope with uncertainty about their health and future prospects.

A feature of all chronic illnesses is that the severity of their effects depends to a large extent on how well individuals manage their condition by making the necessary adjustments to their habits and behaviour. Making these adjustments has other effects on the lives of sufferers and their families, and the extent to which they suffer depends on factors that often have little to do with the original causes of their condition. It is these aspects of sickle cell disease that the remainder of this book is about.

2

Psychosocial Research and Sickle Cell Disease

Sickle cell disease (SCD) is a difficult area in which to conduct properly controlled psychological or psychosocial research. Some of the reasons for this are particular to SCD, whilst others apply equally to other chronic illnesses. The findings of studies may also be difficult to interpret and, even where clear results are obtained, there may be reasons why practical measures are not then implemented. The purpose of this chapter is to provide an overview of the types of study that have been conducted in this area and to consider some of the research issues that should be borne in mind in relation to findings presented in later chapters.

Sickle cell disease has been less well researched from a psychological point of view than some other chronic illnesses. One reason for this is probably that it is by no means the most common; conditions like respiratory allergies, asthma, anaemia, heart disease, and diabetes affect larger numbers of children (Newacheck, McManus, and Fox, 1991), and the psychosocial implications of these conditions have been much more thoroughly researched (Midence, Fuggle, and Davies, 1993). Another is that it has been widely regarded as a 'black disease', which for one reason or another has limited the resources and attention it has received (Anionwu, 1989a). This factor is also partly responsible for the uneasy relationship that has sometimes existed between researchers and their 'subjects'. In many cases those affected by SCD have developed a mistrust of being used as guinea pigs, and have had little faith in the ability of the research establishment to translate findings into concrete measures that would improve their situation (Whitten and Fischhoff, 1974).

Whereas medical research on the genetics and biochemistry of sickle cell disease is now well established, work on the psychosocial aspects of the condition is at a much earlier stage. Preliminary findings have yet to be consolidated into a firm foundation on which more ambitious and detailed research can build, and are very far from being integrated into the wider body of knowledge about the psychology of chronic illness in general or with even

21

wider ranging theories of health behaviour, psychological development, and social adjustment. However, these factors make the field
an exciting area in which to be conducting research, and one in
which there is much progress to be made.

We first describe the different types of study that have been
conducted, dealing with the choices of design and perspective. We
go on to consider more specific issues relating to research of this
kind, such as defining and contacting appropriate samples of
patients from whom to collect data, obtaining realistic measurements of the factors under study, and other more practical problems encountered in research on SCD. Finally, we consider the
interpretation of results, and the translation of research findings
into effective measures to benefit patients.

Different Types of Study

Designing Research

Relationships between sickle cell disease and aspects of patients'
social and psychological functioning can be examined in various
ways in order to answer different types of question. Perhaps the
first question to be considered is the extent to which SCD is in fact
associated with deficits, limitations, or abnormal patterns of
psychosocial adjustment. One way to address this issue is by
collecting information about patients' own experiences by interview or questionnaire and taking the reports at face value. This
approach has the merit of beginning at the beginning, as it were,
with patients' own perceptions of the complications of their condition and of their own needs. Clinical observations made by doctors
in the form of case reports also provide a valuable starting point
for more systematic examinations of psychological or social
aspects of the condition. However, patients' own accounts or the
impressions of doctors may not be sufficient to convince others,
and information collected in this way does not tell us about the
extent to which psychosocial problems or needs are specific to the
group in question. A more rigorous approach is to collect information in a more systematic way, and to make comparisons between
people with SCD and a control group (the 'comparative deficit'
model). Any differences that were found should then be attributable to SCD, and the goal of research of this kind would be to

identify areas of psychological or social functioning in which SCD has a particular effect.

Many studies have compared the educational attainment, psychological status, social adjustment, or other factors related to psychosocial well-being, of people with SCD and those of 'healthy' people. The difficulty here is in selecting a suitable control group, for the way that this is done can influence the results that are obtained. For example, several studies of this kind have produced results suggesting that people with SCD do less well at school, in social activities, and in a variety of other ways, than others. However, when those with SCD are compared with people of the same ethnic and socio-economic groups, differences of this kind are much less commonly found, indicating that, where differences were observed, they were probably caused by demographic and economic factors rather than by SCD *per se*. In children, one way to take account of such factors is to compare those with SCD to their healthy siblings. Another interesting comparison is that between people with SCD and sufferers of other chronic illnesses of the same socio-economic and ethnic background. Differences observed in this case would be specific to SCD, rather than to chronic illness in general.

An alternative to the comparative design is to look at relationships between variables such as illness severity, personality, family interactions, or coping strategies *within* a group of people with SCD (a 'correlational' design). Here the goal is not to identify areas of need or deficits associated specifically with the condition, but to examine factors that are associated with different outcomes among people who have SCD in common. In chronic illness generally it is apparent that functional status and illness severity cannot account for the wide variations in quality of life that have been observed across disease types and between individuals with the same condition (Daniels *et al.*, 1987). The evidence suggests that SCD is no exception; some people fare much better than others and studies of this kind would indicate factors that may assist or facilitate more effective coping or adjustment.

A third type of study to be considered employs a 'before and after' design to examine the effects of particular treatments or interventions. Information is collected about relevant aspects of symptom severity, adjustment, or quality of life, and a comparison is made over time in order to evaluate the efficacy of measures that were introduced during the study period. Interventions that have been examined in this way include behavioural techniques for the management of pain (Zeltzer, Dash, and Holland, 1979; Cozzi,

23

Tryon, and Sedlacek, 1987) and organizational strategies for the delivery of support services (Vichinsky, Johnson, and Lubin, 1982).

In its simplest form this design is actually rather limited, and additional components are needed to be confident that changes observed in the target variables are in fact attributable to the intervention in question (Pocock, 1983). The 'A–B–A' trial, for example, involves removing whatever intervention was introduced to see whether outcome measures return to baseline levels. If they do not, it is possible that improvements apparently due to the novel treatment actually reflected gradual changes over time for reasons unrelated to the trial. A control group allows investigators to differentiate the effects of specific aspects of a new treatment regime from those of more general factors, such as increased attention paid to participants in a trial, or expectations by subjects that things are about to improve. In drug trials, a control group can be given a placebo, but in studies of behavioural or organizational interventions it is more difficult to set up a suitable control. Control subjects might simply be monitored and tested in the same way as those receiving the treatment in question, or might be given a comparable treatment package with a critical ingredient missing. This can be important where novel interventions comprise a combination of potentially effective measures and when simple before and after comparisons would not reveal which component was most important.

Adopting a Perspective

In addition to making a choice about which design to use, the researcher must also select the type of information to be collected for comparison, and this choice will reflect the focus of the study and the questions to be addressed. 'Psychosocial factors' is an umbrella term covering a wide range of possible variables, and SCD can be examined in terms of measures of ability, personality, levels of social and psychological development, interactions with peers and with family members, and many other aspects of psychosocial functioning. By focusing on one aspect, others will necessarily be excluded, for no study can be exhaustive, and a focus of one kind or another cannot be avoided. Lipowski (1971) has identified three broad categories of factors which may be related to adjustment in physical illness. These are: (1) factors related to the disease (e.g. its visibility, duration, severity, and the level of restriction it imposes); (2) those related to the individual (e.g.

personality, abilities, previous experience); and (3) those related to the environment of the patient (e.g. attitudes and responses of family, friends and others). Any of these broad categories could provide a focus for research.

If the focus of a study were too narrow, however, it would not be possible to examine alternative explanations for whatever results were obtained. For example, a study of the academic abilities of children with SCD might show that they scored lower on standardised tests than controls, suggesting that SCD affects levels of intelligence (Swift *et al.*, 1989). The true explanation might be that performance at the tests was influenced not by the disease itself but by enforced absence from school, caused by pain crises or the need to attend hospital, but this would not be revealed by a study whose sole focus was performance on tests of ability. The choice of information to be collected is therefore vital to the accuracy of the picture given by the results, and some authors (Midence *et al.*, 1993, Moise, 1986) have suggested adopting a 'multidimensional approach', taking into account factors such as socio-economic status, marital status, family characteristics, and social support networks in order to obtain the most realistic picture possible of the psychosocial implications of sickle cell disease.

It is also important not to focus exclusively on deficits and problems, but to collect information on more positive responses in order to obtain a more complete picture of adjustment. Much research on chronic illness has focused predominantly on psycho-pathology and dysfunction, with the result that the resilience shown by many families has not been recognized, and information on coping styles and processes has been limited. The work on SCD also conforms to this trend. In many cases strategies can be developed to compensate for limitations and disabilities (Walco and Dampier, 1987), so that a study in which information is collected only on the limitations or deficits imposed by sickle cell may well present an unduly pessimistic picture.

Another way in which a focus can be adopted by a researcher is by linking the study to a particular area of theory. Data might be collected from a particular group of people in order to test some aspect of theory in health psychology or developmental psychology, or to examine the extent to which the psychosocial functioning of people with SCD can be made sense of by applying a theoretical model. In cases of this kind, the choice of data to be collected may well be driven by the requirements of the theory rather than by the need to obtain facts for their own sake.

25

In fact, this type of study is very rare in the field of chronic illness, a situation regretted by Eiser (1990a), who has argued that the psychological functioning of children with chronic illnesses can best be understood by integrating research on the topic with 'stage' theories of psychological development.

Sampling

The way that people are selected to participate in research can clearly influence the results that are obtained. Ideally, findings should be capable of generalization to the widest possible population. Where only a small group of subjects are selected from a small area, or from those who use a particular service or clinic, the results may reflect local factors or characteristics of the group in question rather than more general aspects of the condition. Many of the findings about SCD have been based on studies of relatively small groups, and some of the discrepancies between the results of different studies may be due to differences in the samples used (Lemanek et al., 1986). For example, it has been suggested that health professionals encounter families with more severe problems, whereas studies of families contacted in other ways have found more successful coping (Midence et al., 1993). The most widely representative results would be obtained by inclusive sampling, in which people who may not be in contact with service agencies, and who may therefore be more difficult to recruit into research, are also represented. Ronald Nagel, for example, describes finding two people with SCD during a screening programme in New York. Both were in their late twenties, had never seen a doctor nor saw any reason to, and could not be persuaded to attend the outpatient clinic (Nagel, 1991). Individuals like this, who may be a valuable source of information about living with SCD, would clearly be much more difficult to recruit into research than those who present frequently at hospital with problems related to their condition.

Where there are factors that make it problematic to contact and recruit potential subjects, therefore, there is a danger that those who do participate will not be representative of the general population of people with SCD. The lack of comprehensive care systems and effective community outreach programmes means that people with SCD are often difficult to identify and locate, whilst their lifestyles – sometimes characterized by poverty and stress – mean that co-operation with research may be problematic. In addition, many patients and their families may already feel that they have been 'used' by researchers in the past, and may be unwilling to participate in research from which they perceive no direct benefit to themselves. Moise (1986) has described the patience and perseverance required to collect data from even a relatively small sample of patients.

On the positive side, participation in research can provide an opportunity for those involved to learn more about the condition and about the services and support that may be available to them.

Measurement

This is a critical issue in all social and psychological research, for the reliability of results depends upon the accurate measurement of the characteristics in question. This is especially true when the critical constructs are abstract ones such as adjustment, mental health, personality, or family functioning.

Sources and Forms of Data

Many different aspects of psychosocial functioning have been examined in relation to SCD, and some are more amenable than others to objective and accurate measurement. For example, coping strategies or interpersonal conflicts are very difficult to record accurately, and studies in these areas may have to depend to a large extent upon unsubstantiated self-reporting by subjects. Other factors, such as academic attainment, knowledge about SCD, or performance at standardized tests of ability, can be measured more systematically, with little scope for bias or misrepresentation. In the middle ground are factors such as personality, attitudes, and beliefs, measurement of which can be approached using standardized instruments, but that still depends primarily on information provided by the person. Many such instruments (such as questionnaires, structured interview schedules, and rating scales) are in a continuous state of development and appraisal, and many require modification for use with particular groups of people. In any research of this kind, therefore, one should be prepared to examine critically the ways in which data was obtained, and to look for improvements in the measurement of the

27

characteristics in question. In many areas, work is being conducted on ways of measuring more accurately aspects of SCD such
as severity, pain, and disruption to everyday life.

Quantitative versus Qualitative Data

In order to perform statistical analyses, information must be
coded in numerical form, so that frequencies of concrete events
such as attendances at hospital or absences from work or school
are preferable to qualitative descriptions of symptoms. Similarly,
severity of pain crises may be measured more objectively by
recording levels or frequencies of medication required than by
patient ratings or qualitative data. Other aspects of the condition,
such as family conflicts, social interactions, or participation in
activities, can also be measured in a more objective way by
recording numbers of events of different types, rather than
depending upon patients' own descriptive insights.

However, there is still a valuable role for qualitative data in
scientific research, for many aspects of patients' functioning cannot realistically be captured in numerical form. Coping strategies,
for example, cannot be quantified reliably, and in many cases
patients' own descriptions may provide insights that would not be
revealed by quantitative analyses (e.g. Anionwu and Beattie,
1981). Also, many valuable avenues of scientific investigation
begin with qualitative descriptions of cases and phenomena, so
that qualitative data often serve as the basis for hypotheses that
can then be tested in a more controlled way.

Sources of Measurement Error

There are, broadly speaking, two types of measurement error in
psychological research. The first is random error, or 'noisy' measurement, and is caused by insensitivity of the instrument, or
inherent instability of the construct to be measured. Error of this
kind is in the nature of blurring or fuzziness, so that the information obtained represents only a rough approximation to the real-
ity, with errors in either direction being equally likely. For example, the number of pain crises occurring over a given period may
be only a very rough measure of a person's experience of pain, with
overestimation in some cases and underestimation in others. Some
factors (such as family dynamics) may be inherently problematic
to access by self-report, or may be subject to misattributions or

lack of insight on the part of the subject. Measurement error of this kind may make authentic relationships between variables or differences between groups difficult to detect, especially in small samples.

The second is systematic error, or bias, in which the error of measurement is predominantly in one direction, and which may lead to spurious findings or misleading results. Biases, which may be intentional, accidental, or unconscious, may be introduced by the subject or the researcher. Subjects may feel pressure to respond in particular ways, may wish to give the responses they feel are expected, or may have an agenda of their own (Orne, 1962). Most of these factors could apply equally to researchers, who may allow their own preconceptions, expectations, or hopes to colour the objective collection of data (Rosenthal, 1969). The scope for 'artifacts' of this kind in a field such as SCD is increased by the fact that data can rarely be collected 'blind' to the clinical status of subjects. In a properly controlled clinical trial or psychological investigation (Pocock, 1983), the investigator does not know until afterwards the status or condition of the person from whom they are collecting information. In studies of SCD this is rarely possible, and researchers may be all too clearly aware of which subjects, for example, are SCD patients, and which are 'controls'.

Interpreting Results

The social and psychological aspects of SCD – or any other disease – cannot be examined under controlled conditions in the laboratory. The fact that research must be conducted in the real world means that the results are usually open to more than one interpretation. This is because not all of the factors that were not directly under investigation can be held constant. Certain factors that would be expected to play a role, such as ethnic group or socioeconomic status, can be taken account of by matching subjects and controls, but there is always the possibility that apparently clear relationships between variables might be due to factors which were not taken into account. This is especially true when those being studied have special characteristics that make them unrepresentative of the general population of people with SCD.

29

Complex Relationships between Variables

In many cases several factors may be associated with psychosocial functioning, and where results like this are obtained it may be difficult to identify which are the key variables. For example, children with SCD might score lower than controls on tests of academic achievement. This could be interpreted in different ways: reduced intelligence, lower self-confidence, or less supportive home environments, for example. In fact, the evidence suggests that although SCD was the original cause of differences in achievement, the primary cause is usually reduced attendance at school because of pain crises and other medical complications. If this is true, the disease does not affect academic achievement directly, but has an indirect influence by limiting children's access to schooling (Shapiro *et al.*, 1990). On the basis of such findings, interventions could be designed to support the education of children with sickle cell and compensate for lost days at school. For research to be translated effectively into practical measures it is important that the findings be interpreted accurately, and the potential for this may well depend on the thought that went into designing and carrying out the study; if relevant information was not collected, or was collected unsystematically, then the correct interpretation will be less likely to be arrived at.

Another limitation of research conducted in the real world rather than under laboratory conditions is that where one factor has been shown to be related to another, it is rarely possible to be certain of the direction of causation, that is, which variable is influencing the other. For example, several studies have shown relationships between adjustment to sickle cell and self-concept or self-esteem. This relationship might well operate in either direction; higher self-esteem could assist patients in making the necessary adjustments, better adjustment might enhance self-esteem, or both might influence one another in a complex 'synergistic' relationship. In some cases the nature of the variables make ambiguity about the direction of causation very limited – higher rates of absence from school or work could hardly cause pain crises — but when dealing with relationships between psychological measures there is frequently scope for alternative interpretations. Clear-cut interpretations of results are not always possible, especially where various factors are interrelated. It is relatively simple to list variables that might influence adjustment among people affected by a chronic illness, but much more difficult to predict how they might interact to determine how the person might respond to their condition at any given time. Some attempts to do this have been made for haemophilia and spina bifida (Varni and Wallander, 1988), but not so far for SCD.

One way of dealing with the problem of complex relationships is to use multivariate statistical analyses to examine the independent and interactive relationships among variables. This is rarely possible in small sample studies, for the statistical techniques require large numbers of cases for reliable analyses. They may also make assumptions about the methods of measurement and data collection, so that studies in which sophisticated statistical analyses are to be used should be carefully planned in advance.

Another way is to attempt to control for possible confounding factors by holding them constant. This can be done by screening potential subjects to eliminate factors that are not the main focus of the study. This obviously reduces the number of people from whom data can be collected, which may be a serious practical disadvantage if access to patients is limited to begin with.

Implementing Findings

No single study ever resolves an important psychosocial issue, no matter how large in scale, or how well designed and carried out. In behavioural research a realistic picture emerges only when a body of findings are considered together, and the relative strengths and weaknesses of each study are weighed up along with the results they have produced. Obviously, the most robust findings would be expected to be produced by similar studies in different places, at different times, and with different groups of subjects.

Any given phenomenon can be examined from various points of view, so that where the results of studies using different samples, methods, or theoretical perspectives all point in broadly the same direction, we may be most confident that we are dealing with authentic effects. Apparently divergent findings produced by different studies may begin to make more sense when differences in the ways that the studies were conducted are taken into account. Perhaps those that took certain factors into account tended to give one type of result, whereas those that did not gave another. Results from one group of patients may be different from those of another. This need not mean that the effects observed are unreliable or ephemeral (although they may be). They may be 'interactive'; that is, the relationship between two variables might depend upon some other factor. For example, in the case of diabetes and arthritis, there is evidence that whereas younger children suffer more in terms of school tasks and performance (Rovet, Ehrlick, and Hope, 1987), older children are affected more in areas of social adjustment (Ungerer *et al.*, 1988).

Finally, no one benefits from research unless the means and the will exist to act on the findings. Studies may indicate areas of need or potentially effective new services, but this is only the first step towards improving the level of service provision or implementing new strategies or programmes for the delivery of care and support. Certain measures may be expensive to implement, may be low on the priorities of managers or politicians, or may go against the prevailing ethos. Research can serve a campaigning function in such situations, by amassing the evidence necessary to establish a case for change, and by exerting direct influence on contemporary ways of thinking about health care (Torkington, 1992). All research takes place within a social context and, in applied research on health and illness, the interplay between scientific and social issues is at its most complex. Researchers must usually take the existing order as their starting point, frame the questions they address from what they see around them, and feed their findings back into the political and managerial institutions that have the power to make changes.

3

Pain and Sickle and Cell Disease

In sickle cell disease, body tissue and organs are damaged by oxygen starvation because of obstructed blood flow in the small vessels of the venous system (vaso-occlusion). The nature and severity of such damage is variable, depending upon the extent and the site of sickling, but tissue damage is usually accompanied by pain, which is the most direct and the most distressing aspect of SCD for most sufferers. Pain crises are the principal cause of morbidity amongst patients with SCD (Platt *et al.*, 1991), and account for 90 per cent of SCD-related hospital admissions (Brozovic, Davies, and Brownell, 1987).

Painful episodes restrict the lives of sufferers in various ways, including absence from school or work and disruption to social and family life. Some people with SCD endure extended periods of frequent hospital treatment, although relatively minor episodes, which do not receive medical attention, probably account for most limitations and restrictions to lifestyle in the SCD population as a whole. Shapiro *et al.* (1990) found that among children who were severely affected by SCD, 48 per cent of absences from school were due to pain crises, and that 62 per cent of days lost for this reason were spent at home, without needing hospitalization.

In addition to the practical inconvenience of disruption to everyday life, periodic and unpredictable episodes of incapacitating pain can affect the way people see and feel about themselves, the way they relate to other people, the goals they set themselves, and the way they approach a range of activities and situations. Quality of life between crises may be affected by anxiety about future attacks and the need to follow precautions to minimize the frequency and severity of painful episodes. The experience of pain is always distressing, but if recurrent acute pain is badly managed it can lead to psychological and behavioural problems with effects lasting longer than the pain itself, and there is some concern that SCD pain is sometimes neglected or undertreated by medical staff.

Much of this book is concerned with the ways in which people with SCD respond to recurrent acute episodes of pain. In this chapter we consider the primary characteristics of SCD pain and look at the prevention and management of pain crises. All of the information we present is based on one system or another for recording the frequency or severity of pain, so we begin by considering the issue of assessment and measurement of SCD pain.

Assessment and Measurement of Pain

Pain is essentially a subjective phenomenon, which makes its assessment and measurement problematic for both the clinical care of people in pain and the scientific study of pain. Because pain cannot be inspected directly, clinicians and researchers depend for their information on what people do and say about their pain. Self-reports and behavioural observations form the basis of most attempts to make realistic and reliable assessments of pain. Problems can arise with both forms of data because some of the factors that influence verbal reports or pain behaviour are unrelated or only indirectly related to the physiology or the immediate personal experience of pain.

Incidence

In order to achieve some level of standardization (and to simplify the collection of data), the figures used in many studies of the frequency and distribution of pain crises represent only those occasions when people sought medical help. This may be influenced by various factors including the availability and cost of medical services and their perceived efficacy, which probably vary considerably between different populations. For example, Brozovic and Anionwu (1984) found that far more (93 per cent, compared with 39 per cent) of people with sickle cell anaemia required hospital treatment for painful crises in the UK than in Jamaica. A warmer climate would be expected to reduce the incidence of sickling to some extent, but the difference in numbers treated for pain probably also reflects factors unrelated to physiology, such as the availability of health care provision, methods of pain relief used at home and in hospital, and possibly cultural differences in relation to pain tolerance. Defining a pain episode in this way has also resulted in less attention being paid to pain which did not, for one reason or another, lead to contact with the medical profession.

34

Quality and Intensity of Pain

Accurate and reliable assessment of the quality and intensity of pain is essential for good clinical care, as well as for research into the factors that affect the onset of pain and the effectiveness of management regimes. Most of the factors to be born in mind in assessments of this type are at the personal and interpersonal level, although differences in climate and culture may also influence the experience of pain (Serjeant, 1992). Clinicians usually rely on patients' reports of pain and behavioural observations to assess the severity of pain crises (Walco and Varni, 1991), although the behaviour of the patient in pain and the response of the doctor may be influenced by the two people's preconceptions and expectations of one another (Brookoff, 1991).

A few studies have tried to identify ways of assessing the severity of SCD pain and any negative consequences more objectively (Cameron *et al.*, 1983; Hurtig, Koepke, and Park, 1989), particularly in relation to the assessment of pain in children (McGrath, 1989). However, no universally accepted method for the assessment of paediatric pain exists, and although some physiological parameters have been examined as possible indices of pain intensity, most standardized instruments for the assessment of pain rely heavily on patients' own reports. The McGill Pain Questionnaire (Melzack, 1975), for example, presents people with a range of adjectives describing pain to select from, and has been used to identify the different types of pain sensation and experience associated with various conditions. This method has been adapted and extended in the Varni/Thompson Pediatric Pain Questionnaire (PPQ; Walco and Dampier, 1990) for use with children, by incorporating a visual analogue scale and colour indicators to register the relative intensity of pain, and body figures to indicate its location. Walco and Dampier concluded that SCD pain was comparable in intensity to the very high levels of pain reported in postoperative pain, but tended to be of longer duration.

Pain diaries allow detailed information on pain of all types and severity to be related to factors such as the time and place of painful episodes, and activities and situations that may be important in relation to the onset and the effects of pain. The quality of information gained in this way may vary from person to person, and data may be difficult to standardize, but diaries have been used successfully in one study of the frequency and severity of pain crises that did not necessarily lead to medical attention (Shapiro *et al.*, 1990).

Variations in Frequency, Severity and Type of Pain

Rates of Pain Episodes

Pain crises vary from attacks of mild pain in a joint or bone lasting only a few minutes to very severe and more generalized pain lasting days or weeks and requiring hospital admission and the strongest pain relief. The 'average' SCD patient experiences one or two severe pain crises per year (Varni and Walco, 1988). The majority have very few crises, whereas a significant minority require frequent hospital admissions and have a very disrupted lifestyle. In general, those with SS suffer more than those with SC disease or Sβ thalassaemia, but the pattern of pain varies markedly both between individuals and over time in any one person.

Data from Shapiro et al. (1990) and Brozovic et al. (1987) showed that over half of the pain crises that required medical intervention were experienced by only about one-fifth of the SCD population. Three-quarters of the 260 people with SCD in Walco and Dampier's (1987) study had not been admitted to hospital during the previous 12 months.

In Whitten and Nishiura's (1985) study of pain leading to hospitalization in 348 people with SCD, 26 per cent had not been hospitalized, 55 per cent had been hospitalized between once and five times a year, and 12 per cent had been admitted between six and ten times a year. Slightly fewer crises, but with a similar distribution, were found in the largest and most recent survey of pain frequency. Platt et al. (1991) recorded the frequency of SCD-related pain lasting for over 2 hours and leading to a clinic visit in 3578 people of all ages with SCD in the USA. Those with SS reported a mean of 0.8 crises per year, compared with 0.4 for those with SC disease and SβThalassaemia. Of those with SS, 39 per cent did not report any pain crises, and most reported only one or two, whereas the remaining minority (5%) reported 33 per cent of all the crises.

Changes with Age

Both the incidence of pain and its effects might be expected to change in individuals over time as the condition stabilizes and individuals adopt characteristic patterns of management and response to pain. Brozovic *et al.* (1987) found no differences in rates of hospital admission for pain crises between children of school age and younger children, although Hurtig and White (1986b) found that the numbers of hospital admissions among children fell with increasing age; those aged below 5 years had an average of 2.3 crises per year, compared with 1.2 for those aged between 12 and 16 years. Just as in adults, most crises in childhood are experienced by a minority of individuals. Varni, Walco, and Katz (1989) reported that only twelve out of 260 SCD children experienced over one-half of the total hospital admissions, which ranged from three to 12 a year.

The location of pain alters with age, usually becoming more centralized as the person grows older. In younger children, the arms, legs, and joints are most commonly affected, whereas in older patients pain is increasingly found in the trunk, chest, spine, abdomen, pelvis, or scapulae (Brozovic, Davies, and Henthorn, 1989). Whereas the trunk and visceral organs are often affected in adolescents, pain is more commonly experienced in the spine, pelvis, chest, and abdomen in adults (Davies and Brozovic, 1989).

Between Episodes

During the steady state, that is, the condition outside pain crises, the patient is well but remains anaemic, unable to concentrate urine, sometimes mildly jaundiced, and prone to infections. People may also have the next possible pain crisis on their minds, and may try to behave in such a way as to make it less likely.

Precipitating Factors

Pain crises are often preceded by strenuous physical exertion, dehydration, infection, cold exposure, or unusual stress or trauma, all of which can affect blood flow, although in many instances there is no apparent precipitating factor or event. The most common factors are sudden changes of temperature, cold, exertion, and tiredness (Murray and May, 1988). Exertion can reduce the level of oxygen in the blood and cause acidosis, both of which make red cells more likely to sickle. Dehydration can lead to reduced plasma volume, which interferes with the normal smooth flow in blood vessels by increasing the blood viscosity. Induction of anaesthetics can also cause oxygen depletion. Not all of the mechanisms whereby infections precipitate painful crises are known (Serjeant, 1992), but respiratory infections can cause deoxygenation of sickle haemoglobin, and fever or high temperature also make sickling more likely. Cold exposure can cause vasoconstriction of small vessels and slowing of blood flow.

It is not yet understood how pregnancy *per se* can precipitate pain crises, but this happens most during the last trimester and postpartum phases of pregnancy. Others factors such as emotional stress (Nadel and Portadin, 1977), can also precipitate pain crises, in less predictable ways.

Most patients experience a prodromal phase to the crisis, which is sometimes difficult to describe but alerts the patient that a painful crisis is about to occur and continues until the onset of the crisis itself (Franklin, 1990).

Prevention of Pain

There are a few basic principles and procedures that people with SCD can follow in order to reduce the likelihood of crises, although the frequency, duration, and intensity of pain vary considerably from one individual to another, and good self-management cannot prevent crises entirely. Fluids are important because SCD is associated with impairment of renal concentration, so that by passing large quantities of urine, patients become dehydrated very easily. Dehydration can be prevented by maintaining fluid intake (between 3 and 4 litres for an adult daily). Keeping warm facilitates good circulation, overexertion should be avoided, and periodic rest is strongly advised.

Treatment and Management

Vichinsky, Johnson, and Lubin (1982) have suggested that although there are no simple treatment solutions, appropriate analgesia and supportive counselling are the most effective ways of improving a patient's ability to cope with painful crises. Minor crises are usually managed at home, where prompt self-medication with oral analgesics such as aspirin, paracetamol, or codeine may be sufficient to alleviate the pain. Hospitalization is necessary when the pain is more severe and oral analgesia is ineffective, or when there is a constitutional upset such as breathing difficulties, high temperature (over 38.5 °C), tachycardia, or vomiting.

The three essential aspects to the medical management of painful crises are analgesia, hydration, and identification with treatment of any underlying conditions such as infection. The first priority is prompt and adequate analgesia. The choice of analgesic will depend in part on the local hospital protocol as well as on the type, location, and intensity of pain reported by the patient. A specific pain management protocol for each patient is always recommended (Vichinsky, 1991). The use of opiates is generally required during hospitalization, and most hospitals in Britain use continuous subcutaneous or intramuscular injections of pethidine or morphine (Davies and Brozovic, 1989). Patient-controlled analgesia (PCA) has been a very effective method of administering medication in children and adolescents with SCD (Schechter, Berrin, and Katz, 1988; Holbrook, 1990). PCA systems involve the use of a programmable pump that limits the amount of analgesic administered during a period of time, but allows the patient to control intravenous administration of analgesia as it is needed to eliminate the pain. This is important because pain may come and go during a crisis (Murray and May, 1988), and PCA can break the cycle of pain, anxiety, and sedation often associated with short-acting opiates (Brookoff, 1992).

Patients in crisis may need large amounts of fluids to counter dehydration. If the patient is too ill to drink, fluids can be administered by a fine bore nasogastric tube or intravenously, until there is no further need of parenteral opiates to control the pain (Davies and Brozovic, 1989). Once suitable analgesia and hydration have been achieved, attention needs to be paid to treating the precipitating cause of the pain crisis, and antibiotic therapy is always used in cases of infection. If an underlying cause for the sickling episode is not identified and treated, the pain will persist or recur.

Analgesia and the Risk of Drug Dependence

Some people with SCD require powerful drugs for the control of pain. Most doctors would take the view that avoidable pain is medically unacceptable, and that patients have a right to adequate pain relief. In practice, many feel uneasy about repeated prescriptions of opiates. In a small number of cases, doctors with very liberal prescribing policies have found difficulty in setting limits for their patients (Raphael and Singh, 1984). The medical profession in many countries is also concerned about the possibility of contributing to the scale of the drug problem by creating dependence in patients (Stimmel, 1983; Streltzer, 1980) or by supplying drugs that are diverted onto the black market. Generally, doctors have been encouraged to prescribe opiates for pain associated with malignancy (cancer), but are often cautioned against this for chronic, non-malignant pain (Gildenberg and De Vaul, 1985). Medical fears about dependence are greatest when there is no immediately apparent organic cause for pain or when patients request continued and increased medication (Bell, 1991). In some quarters, excessive caution about prescribing drugs of potential abuse has come close to suspicion and hostility towards chronic pain patients generally. Maruta, Swanson, and Finlayson (1979), for example, have commented that:

> ... because of frequent exposure to drugs of potential abuse, they [patients with chronic pain] may become drug dependent easily, with a subsequent increase in resistance to management of pain. Abuse and dependency should be detected and treated early to minimize some of the difficulties encountered in the treatment-resistance of chronic pain patients.

Opiate dependence would be a problematic complication in SCD because withdrawal could precipitate sickling crises, but the risk of dependence on opiates prescribed for pain is generally overstated, and undermedication for pain is probably a more significant problem than addiction to drugs among people with SCD. There are centres of excellence in the management of SCD, but in many cases misconceptions and lack of expertise among the medical profession appear to have led, or contributed, to significant undertreatment of SCD pain. As Hurtig (1986) has pointed out, 'The medical myth is that pain in SCD is manipulative and can serve to demand attention at best, and drugs at worst'.

Chronic Pain and Addiction

On close inspection, the case for a significant risk of dependence among patients who are prescribed opiates for recurring acute pain would appear to be based more on subjective clinical experience and generalized misconceptions and fears about addiction than on hard evidence. The available data on the prevalence of drug dependence associated with chronic pain show that where there is no previous drug problem history, the risk of dependence developing as a result of treatment with opiates is actually very low.

Porter and Jick (1980) reported a survey in which only four cases of dependence in patients with no previous history of addiction could be found among 12 000 medical inpatients who had been prescribed opiates. Taub (1982) described 313 patients with refractory pain who were maintained on opiates for up to 6 years, among whom the only management problems arose in 16 patients who all had prior drug problem histories. Portenoy and Foley (1986) examined 38 cases in which patients were prescribed opiates on a long term basis for the management of pain. They found that despite having used 'addictive' drugs for up to 7 years, the only cases in which management had become a problem were two patients with a previous history of drug dependence. Other reports of successful long term treatment with opiates for chronic pain include Tennant and Uelman's (1983) study of 22 patients who were maintained on opiates after treatment at a pain clinic had failed, and France, Urban, and Keefe's (1984) report of 16 patients who received low doses of opiates as part of a comprehensive care package. Neither reported any evidence of dependence or problems with management. Haertzen and Hooks (1969) have also shown that long term use of morphine for the relief of pain was not associated with the development of personality traits characteristic of addiction.

There is less reliable evidence on the incidence of drug dependence among people with SCD. Vichinski et al. (1982) noted that there was no incidence of 'drug addiction' among over 600 patients, although Brozovic et al. (1986) reported that, among 101 patients with SCD in Britain, three were 'addicted' to drugs, while another seven were 'drug dependent'. In both of these studies it is unclear exactly what is meant by the terms 'addiction' and 'dependence', and problem drug use may be difficult to define precisely for populations who do have legitimate requirements from time to time for drugs of potential abuse. Payne (1989) reported that among 160 patients at the Sickle Cell Centre in Cincinnati, USA, 14 met more clearly defined criteria for problem drug use.

It would clearly be unrealistic to expect no drug abuse at all among people with SCD when the scale of the drug problem generally is so large. The available evidence suggests that the prevalence of 'drug addiction' among people with SCD is no higher than among the general population. Unfortunately, the belief persists that SCD patients are a problem population and medical staff fear that patients might abuse pain medication and become drug dependent, whereas patients themselves report being more concerned about the side-effects of pain relief than about addiction to medication (Murray and May, 1988).

Undertreatment of Pain

There is a widespread and growing feeling that medical reluctance to use opiates has resulted in significant undertreatment of pain. Marks and Sachar (1973) interviewed and reviewed the charts of 37 inpatients being treated with opiates for pain, and surveyed 102 hospital doctors about their views, beliefs, and practices in relation to opiate prescribing. They found that almost one-third of patients were continuing to experience severe distress, and up to two-thirds were being undertreated for their pain. Many of the doctors underestimated effective dose ranges and overestimated the duration of action of analgesics. Many also exaggerated the dangers of addiction, and those who did so were more likely to prescribe lower doses of pain relief.

Undertreatment of pain can lead to the very types of problem behaviour that doctors are trying to avoid. Weissman and Haddox (1989) described the case of a young inpatient who was making repeated requests for increased pain medication for a variety of complaints unrelated to his primary condition (acute leukaemia). Medical and nursing staff were suspicious that the pain he was reporting was not real and that he was becoming addicted to the medication, but a review of the case revealed that his apparently 'manipulative' behaviour was a result of undertreatment of his pain. When trust breaks down between a doctor and a patient in pain because the doctor does not accept the patient's report of pain, the patient must resort to manipulative or exaggerated pain behaviour to obtain adequate analgesia. This can then be construed by the doctor as evidence of dependency.

There is considerable evidence on the effects of unnecessary suffering on patients due to undertreatment of pain. Most comes from studies of cancer patients, for SCD has been neglected by research of this kind, but there is no reason to suppose that people with SCD should respond to pain any differently from those with other painful conditions. Cleeland (1984) has described how unrelieved pain increases sensitivity to other physical symptoms and affects basic functions such as appetite and sleep, as well as fostering loss of trust, reduced self-esteem, and feelings of anger and isolation. Marks and Sachar (1973) found that among inpatients whose pain was inadequately treated, sleeping difficulty was the most commonly reported problem, followed by loss of concentration, anxiety, depression, irritability, and crying. Ronald Melzack (1990) has pointed out that, 'Pain impedes recovery from injury and, in the weakened or the elderly, may actually make the difference between life or death'.

There is little hard evidence on the extent of undertreatment of pain for SCD, but very strong grounds for suspecting that SCD pain is among the most neglected and undertreated of any pain in medicine. Alarming numbers of doctors know too little about SCD or about the treatment of pain, so that 'drug-seeking' behaviour is often ascribed to people in genuine pain (Brookoff, 1992). The episodic and unpredictable nature of SCD pain means that people in crisis often suffer considerably before obtaining medical help. Many doctors are doubly reluctant to prescribe opiates on an outpatient basis, which would allow some of those affected to treat their pain promptly at home. In hospital, inappropriate drug regimes often mean that patients either suffer when the duration of action of drugs given 'by the clock' is underestimated, or must convince a member of staff of their need for 'prn' (as needed) medication. As Brookoff (1991) has pointed out, 'prn' as applied to the treatment of pain translates as 'too late'. Patient controlled analgesia (PCA) and prescribing opiates for use at home if needed following discharge probably have less potential for abuse and management difficulties than is often assumed. A more responsive use of analgesics eliminates the need for manipulative pain behaviour, so it can help to foster more positive attitudes and behaviours among medical staff towards people with SCD (Brookoff, 1992), from which all concerned benefit. PCA can also help to prevent patients feeling drugged, which is often reported with oral morphine (McQuay, 1989). The fact that people with SCD are usually black also means that they are vulnerable to racial prejudice and stereotypical attitudes among some medical staff in relation to drug abuse.

Finally, it is worth bearing in mind that even the few patients who do have an authentic drug problem should be entitled to treatment when they are in pain. Opiate-addicted people with SCD would be problematic cases to treat effectively for pain or for addiction, but as Payne (1989, p. 202) has pointed out:

> There is a clear need to develop an interdisciplinary model of care for patients who abuse drugs, but who nevertheless require medical attention (which might include the legitimate use of opioids) for the management of acute or chronic severe pain in whom the abstinence model is not appropriate.

Behavioural Approaches to Pain Management

Various behavioural techniques including biofeedback, hypnosis, imagery, reinforcement, and electrical stimulation exist for the management and control of pain as alternatives or adjuncts to treatment with drugs (Fordyce, 1976). Usually they are resorted to by patients who have found drugs ineffective or whose doctors are reluctant to prescribe adequate medication. They are also attractive to those who prefer not to use drugs or who want to minimize the doses they require, and those who have experienced adverse drug reactions.

Behavioural methods would also be preferable for those who wish to achieve maximum autonomy in the control of their pain, as they represent a step away from the confines of medicine, with emphasis on prevention and management rather than straightforward relief of pain. Disadvantages include the possibility that behavioural methods would be less effective than drugs in the control of more severe pain. Some methods require a certain level of training or competence and, in some cases, specialized equipment or teamwork, so that they would not be suitable for every person. Behavioural techniques can, however, be used in conjunction with conventional analgesia to help to reduce the amount and frequency of drugs needed, and to give patients with pain a more active role in the management of their condition.

Psychological factors in the treatment of pain crises are often overlooked (Walco and Varni, 1991), and evidence on the effectiveness of such methods for the control of pain in SCD is limited to the results of a few studies of techniques such as self-hypnosis, biofeedback, and transcutaneous electrical nerve stimulation (TENS). Most of these were simple comparisons of symptoms and treatment needs before and after a particular management strategy was introduced, without control groups of patients who did

44

not use the method in question or who used it in a different way. In such studies it is not possible to assess the extent to which apparent improvements were due to 'placebo' effects, which might arise from expectations that the method would work or benefits due to the attention and consideration given to patients taking part in a trial. Nor is it possible in every case to be confident about exactly how a treatment was effective, or which component of a package of measures was the active one. For example, muscular relaxation, meditation, hypnosis, and biofeedback have all been shown to be effective in reducing distress in children undergoing painful treatment after burn injuries (Elliot and Olson, 1983), but it is not clear which methods are most effective for particular types of patient, types of pain, and treatment circumstances. There is a need in this area for studies that compare different pain management techniques so as to enable clinicians to tailor pain management according to the needs of individual patients with SCD.

Zeltzer, Dash, and Holland (1979) recorded hospitalizations and analgesic needs of two 20-year-old men with SCD before and after they were trained to use self-hypnosis to induce relaxation and images of their blood vessels dilating to allow sickled cells to pass through. Both young men had a history of severe pain and frequent but unsatisfactory medical treatment, which was complicated in one case by 'problematic' drug use. Physiological biofeedback confirmed that peripheral vasodilation did take place during hypnosis, but the most striking aspect of the results was the reduced need for conventional pain relief. The numbers of emergency room visits made by the two patients fell from 54 to 2, and their hospital admissions fell from 16 to 0, during the 4 months after they began using hypnosis compared with the previous 12 months. Use of narcotic drugs fell significantly in one case and was eliminated altogether in the other. One limitation of the study was that the two patients were monitored for only a short period after training in self-hypnosis, so it is not clear to what extent the dramatic improvements would be sustainable over the long term. However, secondary benefits in the areas of social activity, education, and employment were also noted for both young men. Hypnosis may not be effective for everyone; the authors noted that young people generally make better hypnotic subjects, and hypnosis is probably most effective when used at the very onset of pain, rather than when it is already well established.

Thomas *et al.* (1984) combined hypnosis with thermal biofeedback, relaxation training, and cognitive strategies in a package of behavioural pain control techniques taught to 15 adults with SCD aged between 22 and 35 years. The numbers of emergency room visits fell by 32 per cent, hospital admissions by 31 per cent, time spent in hospital by 50 per cent, and analgesic use by 29 per cent compared with pretraining periods, although it was not possible to identify which aspects of the behavioural programme were most effective.

Cozzi *et al.* (1987) focused specifically on the effects of biofeedback in a study of eight younger people (aged between 10 and 20 years) with SCD, who were given 12 weekly training sessions in the use of electromyographic (EMG) and thermal (digital) feedback. EMG and finger temperature data indicated that feedback was associated with significant physiological changes, and reported headaches, pain intensity, and frequency of analgesia use fell significantly over the 12-week training period. However, 6 months after the training, the numbers of emergency room visits and hospital admissions had not fallen significantly by comparison with the previous 6 months, and the authors suggested that the usefulness of the treatment approach may be limited to milder forms of pain crises.

In the only placebo-controlled trial of a behavioural technique for the control of pain in SCD, Wang *et al.* (1985) examined the efficacy of transcutaneous electrical nerve stimulation (TENS) in a double-blind study of 22 patients between 12 and 27 years of age. ('Double-blind' refers to the fact that neither subjects nor experimenters were told which patients received the full TENS treatment. A placebo-controlled design is possible for a technique like this because patients can be taken through the full treatment procedure without the current being switched on.) The results showed that although about three-quarters of the patients reported finding the treatment useful, there was no significant difference in pain ratings between the TENS and the placebo groups.

Organizational Strategies

There is evidence that a psychosocial approach to pain management within a multidisciplinary team can provide more effective management of SCD pain and less use of medical services. Vichinsky *et al.* (1982) used a psychosocial programme involving support groups, self-hypnosis, psychosocial assessment and follow-up, psychotherapy, a 24-hour hot-line, and home visits by nurses. The programme was implemented in a flexible way, with packages of support tailored to individual needs, and led to a fall in emergency visits of 58 per cent and in hospital admissions of 48 per cent, compared with a previous period.

A near-universal consensus exists among those working most closely with SCD that close integration of services for the assessment and provision of a wide range of needs is the essential element in effective care for those in pain (Walco and Dampier, 1987; Vichinsky, 1991). The disciplines involved should cover expertise in the administration of analgesia and familiarity with behavioural or psychological aspects of SCD pain. Closer involvement by the affected person in the management of their own pain is probably one of the key components of any behavioural strategy for pain management, and this can be promoted by interdisciplinary support from medical and non-medical staff providing counselling, information, and analgesia where necessary. The family of the affected person may also benefit from support during periods of pain (Wethers, 1982; Shapiro, 1989).

Murray and May (1988) have suggested that education of patients and their families about how to avoid crises may lead to a decrease in the number and severity of painful episodes. Those working with people affected by SCD would also benefit from more, and more accurate, information about the individual and social factors related to SCD pain, and more research is needed in this area. Better record-keeping about the incidence and treatment of pain in SCD would provide useful data for such studies, as well as helping carers and sufferers to approach individual problems of pain management in the most effective way.

4

Sickle Cell Disease in Childhood and Adolescence

Many of the psychologically significant processes and events of childhood, such as education, socialization, and the formation of characteristic ways of responding to situations and people have important consequences for adult life. The way we feel about ourselves and about the world is established for the first time in early childhood, and although these feelings change throughout life, the early period of learning and development is a critical influence on our psychological careers. For a person with a chronic illness such as sickle cell disease this is doubly true, for such conditions often impose lifelong limitations and restrictions to which the individual must learn to adapt, so that experiences of the illness and responses to it early in life can influence the long-term adjustment and quality of life of affected people. The child with SCD will have additional knowledge and skills to acquire if he or she is to be able to take responsibility for the management of their condition when the time comes, and he or she must also come to terms emotionally with the condition and any limitations it imposes.

The various tasks and challenges that childhood presents to everyone are also likely to be made more difficult by SCD. The restrictions and limitations that may be imposed by the illness will be felt at first hand for the first time, and comparisons with healthy peers will bring home to the child that he or she is different from other children. In infancy the child is completely dependent on others for its health care, and may suffer because its carers do not yet know of, or know enough about, the condition. The baby with SCD, for example, may be in pain for reasons that have not been identified and that the infant cannot communicate to others. In early childhood, spontaneous play and interaction with peers may be disrupted by episodes of pain and sickness, and relationships with parents and siblings may be coloured by the child's condition. In later childhood, SCD may hamper progress in education and the achievement of independence from the family. The emotional upheaval of the teenage years may be compounded by effects of SCD, such as delayed puberty and growth, and ambitions and aspirations for adult life may have to be revised in the light of limitations imposed by SCD.

It is also worth remembering that for some children with SCD (a minority now) childhood is more than an important period – it is the whole of their lives, for around 11 per cent of children with SCD (15 per cent of those with SS) do not survive into adulthood (Leikin et al., 1989). Even among those who do go on to live long and relatively healthy lives, uncertainty and anxiety about the future are among the features of SCD that must be coped with in childhood.

This chapter examines first the extent to which SCD is in fact associated with problems of psychological and social adjustment and development. We then go on to look at factors that seem to influence the extent to which individuals with SCD are adversely affected, including the severity of the condition and aspects of personality and family environment. Finally, we consider the impact of SCD on school activities and performance.

Studies of Psychological Adjustment and Cognitive Ability

There is now a growing body of knowledge about the social and psychological effects of various chronic illnesses in childhood (see Eiser, 1990a; 1990b for recent reviews). Most of the work on these aspects of SCD has also focused on children rather than adults, but the scope of studies in this field has generally been limited to rather gross comparisons between groups of people or between disease-related variables and indices of adjustment. There are no longitudinal studies tracing the development of affected individuals over extended periods, and few findings that have attempted to relate adjustment in SCD to more general processes of psychological and social development, or to specific ethnic and cultural factors that might be expected to modify or influence the impact of chronic illness in early life. Also, very few of the findings come from research conducted in Britain, for social science in this country has been slow to respond to the challenge of SCD by comparison with, for example, the United States, where most of the studies we report were carried out. The extent to which findings might generalize from one geographical population to another is therefore an additional factor to be considered in evaluating the significance and relevance of different results.

Three broad categories of study are considered separately here. The first is of simple descriptive studies in which information was collected from children, their parents, or their teachers, without any attempt to make comparisons with other groups or to look for systematic relationships between factors. The second is of comparative studies in which children with SCD were compared with healthy children using a variety of standardized or semistandardized psychological instruments. The third is of correlational studies in which different factors relevant either to SCD or to aspects of psychological adjustment were related to one another in order to identify characteristics of the condition, or of the child, which might increase or decrease the risk of psychological problems or maladjustment during development. The main features of those studies in the second and third categories are summarized in Table 1.

Descriptive Studies

Studies of psychosocial aspects of SCD relevant to childhood and adolescence conducted in the UK include a small-scale study on the experiences of a group of parents in Brent (Anionwu and Beattie, 1981), interviews with four schoolchildren with SCD in South London (Patterson, 1980), a survey of the experiences of families in Newham (Black and Laws, 1986), and two studies of the coping difficulties reported by mothers and children with SCD (Midence *et al.*, 1992a,b). All showed a range of positive and negative experiences and responses that were captured by verbatim reports made by the participants and descriptive statistics about the extent to which SCD affected children's lives in different ways.

In New York, Conyard, Krishnamurthy, and Dosik (1980) studied 21 adolescents with SCD by obtaining ratings from hospital social workers, parents, and school teachers about each child in relation to social behaviours including leadership qualities, mental responses and communication, relationships with peers and teachers, adjustment, attendance and participation in school activities, independence, reactions to suggestions, and neatness. Although no statistical analysis was applied to the data, the results

Table 1

Psychosocial studies of children and adolescents with SCD

Study	Sample	Controls	Country	Measures	Results
Kumar et al. (1976)	29 SS (12–18 years)	26 healthy controls	US	California Test of Personality; Piers–Harris Self Concept Scale; General Anxiety Scale for Children	No significant differences. Self concept and anxiety scores lower than controls
Lemanek et al (1986)	30 SCD (17 SS, 8 SC, 5 SβThal) (6–16 years)	30 healthy controls	US	Piers–Harris Children's Scale; Children's Depression Inventory; Behaviour Rating Profile; WISC-R; Child Behaviour Checklist; parents' discipline methods/ knowledge questionnaire	No significant differences between groups. Psychosocial problems may be due to low socio-economic status in SCD children
Morgan and Jackson (1986)	24 SS (12–17 years)	24 healthy controls (matched for age, sex, race, and socio-economic status)	US	Body Cathexis Scale; Children's Depression Inventory; Social Competence Scales of Child Behaviour Profile; Anxiety–Withdrawal Scale of Revised Behaviour Problem Checklist; Structured interview	SS adolescents less satisfied with their bodies and had more symptoms of depression than controls. SS group also spent less time in social/non-social activities

Study	Sample	Controls	Country	Measures	Findings
Akenzua (1990)	204 SS (6–16 years)	208 controls from out-patient clinic	Nigeria	Pediatric Checklist; psychosocial questionnaires	Psychosocial disorders more frequent in SS sample
Iloeje (1991)	84 SCD (6–13 years)	84 healthy classroom peers	Nigeria	Rutter Scales (parents and teachers); Draw a Person Test	Higher levels of psychiatric disturbances amongst SCD children than controls
Hurtig (1986)	12 SCD (8–16 years)	No controls	US	WISC-R; California Test of Personality; Children's Behavioural Profile; Family Environment Scale; Norwicki–Strickland Scale; Piers–Harris Scale	Adolescents with more frequent hospitalizations had lower self-esteem, external locus of control and poorer personality and social adjustment
Hurtig et al. (1989)	70 SCD (8–16 years)	No controls	US	Reports (parents and teachers); WISC-R; Piers–Harris Self-Concept Scale; California Test of Personality; Child Behaviour Checklist	Severity of condition did not predict or affect psychosocial adjustment. Problems in adjustment were most common among older boys
Hurtig and White (1986a)	50 SCD (8–16 years)	No controls	US	WISC-R; California Test of Personality; Child Behaviour Profile; Norwicki–Strickland Locus of Control Scale; Piers–Harris Self-Concept Scale	More behaviour problems and social maladjustment among male adolescents

Table 1 (Cont.)

Study	Sample	Controls	Country	Measures	Results
Hurtig and Park (1989)	33 SCD (12–17 years)	No controls	US	Child Behaviour Profile; Child Behaviour Checklist; Family Environment Scale; Family Inventory of Life Events	Children's scores were low but fell within Achenback's normative sample. Family dynamics were important factors in reducing behavioural problems
Moise (1986)	33 SS (8–16 years)	No controls	US	Norwicki–Strickland Scale; Family Environment Scale; Piers–Harris Scale; California Test of Personality; Child Behaviour Profile	Better adjustment was associated with internal locus of control, and more positive self-concept
Chodorkoff and Whitten (1963)	19 SS (4–14 years)	19 siblings (6–13 years)	US	Stanford–Binet IQ; WISC; Draw-a-Person Test	No significant differences between groups
Gilbert (1970)	30 SS (school-aged)	67 healthy children (51 siblings)	US	Stanford–Binet IQ; Goodenough–Harris Drawing Test; Digit span; Bender Gestalt Visual–motor Test	SS children scored lower on the Stanford–Binet and digit span test

| Swift et al. (1989) | 21 SS (7–16 years) | 21 siblings | US | WISC-R subscales; Detroit test of learning aptitude; Beery Developmental Test of visual–motor skills; Social Competence scales of Child Behaviour Checklist; reading and mathematics scales of the Woodcock–Johnson Psychoeducational Battery; measures of illness severity | SS children scored lower on tests of ability, but scores were not significantly associated with measures of illness severity |
| Fowler et al. (1986) | 28 SCD (school-aged) | Clinic sample of healthy children matched for age, sex, and race | US | Visual–motor integration test; WISC-R subscales; School data; measures of illness severity | SCD children scored below average on tests of ability, and had more problems at school than controls. Ability scores were not correlated with measures of illness severity |

SβThal, sickleβThalassaemia; SC, SC disease; SCD, sickle cell disease; SS, sickle cell anaemia; WISC, Wechsler Intelligence Scale for Children; WISC-R, Wechsler Intelligence Scale for Children-Revised.

presented a generally gloomy picture, suggesting that many of the young people were prone to isolation, dependence, and withdrawal from relationships with their peers in school as well as with their families. Other problems that were noted in some cases included emotional difficulties, poor self-image, depression, anxiety, poor verbalization, and preoccupation with death.

Comparative Studies

The results of descriptive studies set out the general range of symptoms and characteristics among which controlled studies have sought links with SCD in children. Factors under investigation in more scientific research are often given names which reflect concern about objectivity and precision, but the concepts behind the jargon usually correspond to aspects of children's views and feelings about themselves and their behaviour in relation to others. Other constructs under investigation relate to more basic intellectual functioning, as measured by standard tests of general intelligence or specific cognitive abilities.

Social and Psychological Adjustment

Much of the evidence of psychosocial maladjustment in children with SCD has come from studies in Nigeria. Akenzua (1990) used a revised version of the Paediatric Symptoms Checklist (PSC), a screening questionnaire for psychosocial disorders, to look at emotional disturbances in 204 children with sickle cell anaemia (SS) and 208 children without SCD, all aged between 6 and 16 years. The SS group registered a mean score of 18, compared with 13 for the control group; 30 children with SCD (15 per cent), compared with only two of the control group (1 per cent) scored at or above the cut-off point of 28 for detecting psychosocial problems.

Iloeje (1991), also in Nigeria, used Rutter's Behaviour Questionnaires (completed by parents and teachers), and the Draw-a-Person test (DAPT), completed by the children, to look at psychiatric morbidity and intellectual functioning in 84 children with SCD and 84 healthy controls. The Draw-a-Person test showed no differences in intellectual performance between the groups, but the incidence of psychiatric morbidity in the SCD sample was 26 per cent for the parents' scale and 22 per cent for the teachers' scale, compared with 5 per cent and 6 per cent, respectively, for the controls. Boys with SCD were rated higher than girls for psychiatric morbidity, and older children higher than younger ones.

Results like these would suggest that children with SCD are at significantly higher risk than their peers of psychological disorders, and the samples concerned are larger than in any comparable studies, but two factors make the findings difficult to interpret from a European or North American point of view. First, there is evidence that levels of emotional disturbance as measured by standardized Western questionnaires are relatively high among the general Nigerian population. Jegede *et al.* (1990), for example, found even higher rates of psychological and emotional disturbance than those reported by Iloeje and Akenzua. Second, we know less about knowledge, attitudes, and levels of service provision in relation to SCD in Nigeria, compared with those in the UK or the US.

A third study indicating problems in adjustment associated with SCD looked at older children in the USA. Morgan and Jackson (1986) measured body satisfaction, depression, and social withdrawal in 24 young people aged between 12 and 17 years with sickle cell anaemia and 24 healthy young people of the same age, sex, race, and socio-economic status (SES). The instruments used for assessment included the Body Cathexis Scale (BCS), the Children's Depression Inventory (CDI), the Social Competence Scales of the Child Behaviour Profile, the Anxiety–Withdrawal Scale of the Revised Behaviour Problem Checklist, and a structured interview to allow subjects to report on relevant areas in their own words. As the authors had predicted, the results indicated that the SCD group were less satisfied with their bodies, showed more symptoms of depression and social withdrawal, and spent less time in social activities than the control group. Retarded growth and delayed puberty, limited physical capacity, and academic underachievement were among the factors that the investigators considered might predispose teenagers with SCD to psychological maladjustment by increasing any difficulty they might have in coping with the normal developmental tasks of adolescence.

Other very similar types of study, however, have failed to find comparable differences in psychological adjustment between children with SCD and healthy controls, or have indicated better adjustment among children with SCD. Kumar *et al.* (1976) looked at personal and social adjustment, anxiety, and self-concept in 29 adolescents with sickle cell anaemia and a control group without any chronic illness, in Los Angeles. No differences in personal and social adjustment (assessed with the California Test of Personality) were found, but the SCD group scored significantly lower than controls (indicating better adjustment) on the General Anxiety Scale for Children and the Piers–Harris self-concept scale. The authors did not attempt to explain the findings, but it may be significant that the young people with SCD were selected from a 'well patient' group, who had not been hospitalized during the previous 3 months. This type of person with SCD might be expected to be least likely to manifest psychological problems, although the results underline the fact that SCD need not always be associated with psychological problems, and in some circumstances might even contribute to enhanced psychological well being.

Another study that found no significant differences between young people with SCD and healthy controls, and which focused more on behavioural characteristics, was conducted in Louisiana, by Lemanek et al. (1986). They compared 30 children and adolescents with SCD (17 with sickle cell anaemia, eight with SC disease, and five with Sβ Thalassaemia) with a control group of 30 healthy young people using a battery of measures including the Piers–Harris Children's Scale, the Children's Depression Inventory (CDI), the Behaviour Rating Profile (BRP), the Wechsler Intelligence Scale for Children-Revised (WISC-R), the Child Behaviour Checklist (CBCL, completed by parents and doctors of the children), and the Parent Discipline Methods/Knowledge Questionnaire (DM/K), supplemented by interviews with the parents and medical data. There was no evidence of higher levels of problem behaviour among the SCD group, although both groups manifested behavioural problems at the upper end of the 'normal' range, which the authors attributed to social and economic factors associated with poverty and minority status, rather than factors related to illness.

Intelligence and Ability

Another series of studies used measurements of IQ and specific cognitive abilities to examine the possibility that SCD is associated with subtle neurological defects that might affect intellectual functioning even in the absence of overt neurological complications. Several of these studies appeared to show deficits in intelligence and ability among children with SCD but, for various reasons, the findings are difficult to interpret clearly.

Fowler *et al.* (1986) tested 28 school-aged children with SCD and a healthy, matched sample on the WISC-R ability scales and a visual–motor integration test. They found that, on the test of visual–motor integration, the children with SCD scored 42 months below the chronological age norms for the test. They also scored relatively low on several scales of the WISC-R. The control group performed better on these tests, but it was unclear whether the apparently low scores of the children with SCD occurred as a direct result of the illness, or whether they were due to other factors such as social deprivation and reduced access to schooling. There was, however, no relationship between test data and measures of illness severity such as numbers of days hospitalized, numbers of crises, and limitations to physical activity however, which might suggest that SCD was not the immediate cause of relatively low ability scores.

The first direct comparison between children with SCD and healthy controls in terms of IQ was made by Chodorkoff and Whitten (1963), in Detroit. They tested 19 children with sickle cell anaemia aged between 4 and 14 years, and 19 sibling controls, using the Stanford–Binet test for children under 8 years old and the Wechsler Intelligence Scale for Children (WISC) for those over 8 years of age. The scores of both groups were generally low to average, but there were no significant differences between the two groups. However, the fact that different tests were used for the two age groups limited the scope of the statistical analysis because the performance of children of different ages could not be compared directly.

Two better-controlled studies have found differences in intelligence test performance between children with SCD and controls. Gilbert (1970) compared 30 school-aged children with sickle cell anaemia to a control group of 67 children of similar age, including 51 siblings of the children with SS. Of the control group, 42 had sickle cell trait and 25 had normal haemoglobin. The children were tested on a range of measures of intelligence and ability, including the Stanford–Binet test, the Goodenough–Harris Drawing test, the Digit Span test (a measure of short-term memory), and other tests of visual, auditory, and motor abilities. The children with sickle cell anaemia scored significantly lower than the controls on the Stanford–Binet test and the digit span test. On the Stanford–Binet test, the SS group average was 79.5, compared with 89.1 and 89.3 for the sickle cell trait and normal haemoglobin groups, respectively. On the digit span test, the SS group recalled 7.6 numbers on average, compared with 8.8 and 9.3, respectively, for the two control groups.

Swift *et al.* (1989) looked at cognitive functioning in relation to measures of illness severity among 21 children with sickle cell anaemia, and made comparisons with 21 healthy siblings aged between 7 and 16 years. Cognitive abilities were assessed by examining scores on specific subscales of the Wechsler Intelligence Scale for Children (WISC-R) and other tests of memory, visual–motor skills, reading and mathematical ability, academic achievement, and social competence. The results showed that the children with sickle cell anaemia scored approximately 1 standard deviation below the controls on most of the subscales of the WISC and the other measures of cognitive ability, but not on the tests of academic achievement and social competence. The authors interpreted the results as evidence that SCD was associated with some degree of cognitive impairment even in the absence of neurological complications. However, test scores did not appear to be related to measures of illness severity. IQ was significantly correlated with frequency of vaso-occlusive and splenic sequestration crises, but most of these associations were due to one subject who recorded an IQ in the moderately retarded range and who also had the only splenic sequestration crisis of the sample, and more vaso-occlusive crises than any other child. In the group as a whole, no measures of disease severity were associated with cognitive outcome.

Summary of the Results of Comparative Studies

The evidence on SCD and psychosocial adjustment is mixed, with some studies providing evidence of behavioural or psychological problems, especially in adolescents, and others pointing to great variability among children with SCD and showing that considerable numbers enjoy good psychological health. General conclusions are made more difficult by the fact that the studies were conducted in different countries; used different criteria for the selection of subjects; and involved various different methods for the assessment of psychological adjustment, some of which were based primarily on information obtained from the subjects themselves and some more on the observations of others. But the main limitation of this approach is that, even where problems are found among children with SCD, group comparisons do not allow the factors that might predispose those children who do seem to suffer psychologically to be identified. Any psychosocial interventions to prevent or treat psychological problems among children with SCD would need to be targeted at those factors. It is for this reason that some researchers (e.g. Hurtig and White, 1986b) have pointed out that comparing chronically ill children as a group with controls does not provide information about variables associated with positive psychological functioning and adjustment in a particular chronic illness, and have called for more 'within-group' studies to identify those children who are at higher risk and specify the factors that are associated with psychological maladjustment.

In terms of intelligence and ability, two studies of the three that compared children with SCD to controls found lower scores on standardized tests among the SCD groups. The studies concerned excluded children with a history of neurological problems, but one interpretation of the findings is that the observed performance deficits were attributable to subtle neurological damage caused by vaso-occlusion in the central nervous system, even in the absence of overt neurological complications. However, various factors would be expected to influence performance on tests of intelligence, including familiarity with the types of task involved, so that differences in the educational experiences of children with and without SCD might also contribute to differences in performance on IQ tests.

If subtle neurological damage was the cause of intellectual deficits in children with SCD, one might expect greater deficits among those who were more severely affected by SCD, whereas in those studies where IQ was related to illness severity, no significant relationships were found. Subtle neurological damage caused by vaso-occlusion might also be expected to affect particular abilities, reflecting damage to specific areas of the brain, rather than generalized intelligence. The site of the damage and the corresponding deficit in performance would then be expected to vary from one individual to another. Ability testing of this kind might therefore be more appropriate for in-depth assessment of individuals than for aggregated comparisons between groups. In cases where neurological effects of this kind were suspected, test performance over a range of specific abilities could be related to the results of physiological investigations, using modern techniques of brain scanning and imaging to identify the sites of any neural damage.

Correlational Studies

Given that some children with SCD may be at risk of developing psychological problems, but that others apparently are not, the most useful studies in the area of psychological adjustment are those that go beyond comparisons between groups of sick and healthy people to consider individual differences in adjustment among children with SCD. The most important question is why some children with SCD cope well whereas others with the same condition experience social and psychological difficulties. Finding a satisfactory answer to this means identifying particular factors related to the illness, the child, their family, or their environment that place some children and adolescents at increased risk. There is also a need to examine more closely the nature of the problems encountered by children and adolescents with SCD, and to identify the successful strategies for coping and adaptation which are employed by some young people with SCD.

Illness Severity, Age, and Sex

Most of the work on the relationships between indices of the severity of SCD in medical terms and the psychological status of the sufferer was conducted by Anita Hurtig and colleagues at the University of Illinois at Chicago in the late 1980s. Hurtig (1986) reported on a preliminary study of 12 SCD patients aged from 8 to 16 years. This was part of a 5-year project to assess personal and social adjustment as a function of illness variables such as the type of sickle cell disease; the child's age at diagnosis; the frequency and intensity of pain crises; and whether or not strokes, growth retardation, or enuresis (bedwetting) were involved. Information about a range of social and behavioural characteristics was obtained for each patient, including measures of personality, intelligence, family and social functioning, and performance at school.

The data were analysed separately for children above and below the age of 12, and showed that different illness-related variables seemed to be important at different ages. In the younger group, the type of disease seemed to be most closely related to adjustment. Children with SC disease had higher scores for IQ, self-esteem, and levels of social functioning than those with sickle cell anaemia, and were rated by their parents as performing better in school and having fewer absences. Among the older children, aspects of severity that cut across illness types seemed to play a larger role. Those with more frequent pain crises, hospital admissions, and emergency room visits appeared to have lower self-esteem and IQ, poorer social competence and adjustment, more behavioural problems, and a more 'external' locus of control. ('Locus of control' refers to the extent to which positive and negative events are attributed to internal (personal) or external (environmental) factors.) However, the most important factor in the adjustment of adolescents was the age at which a diagnosis of SCD was made (a measure of the duration of illness), which appeared to be associated with most of the psychological and behavioural measures. Hurtig concluded that:

> ... the earlier the diagnosis is made in the adolescent's life, the more likely it is that intelligence, self-esteem, personality, and total adjustment will be reduced, and that locus of control will be external.

However, a later, and larger, study of illness severity and psychosocial adjustment failed to reproduce those findings. Hurtig *et al.* (1989) looked again at the way that numbers of hospital admissions and emergency room visits, frequency and severity of pain crises, and duration of illness were related to the same range of psychological and social variables as in Hurtig's (1986) study. Seventy people with sickle cell anaemia participated, aged between 8 and 16 years. The results this time showed that factors like the age and sex of the patients were better predictors of psychosocial adjustment than were measures of illness severity. The highest levels of behavioural problems and psychological maladjustment were among the older boys, who appeared to be affected by SCD to a greater extent than either younger boys or older girls, irrespective of the duration of illness, patterns of pain crises, and levels of medical care needed.

Similar findings were reported by Hurtig and White (1986a), who looked at 50 young people with SCD, aged between 8 and 16 years. Using measures of adjustment including the revised Wechsler Intelligence Scale for Children (WISC-R), the California Test of Personality (CTP), the revised Child Behaviour Profile (CBP), the Norwicki-Strickland Locus of Control Scale, the Piers–Harris Self-concept Scale, and structured interviews with the children and their parents, they found that the boys were doing less well generally than the girls, and that their problems tended to be in the areas of social and behavioural adjustment, rather than intellectual or personality development.

Illness severity therefore appears not to be associated reliably with adjustment among children with SCD. Only one of the series of studies conducted by Hurtig and her colleagues found evidence of such a relationship, and this was the smallest of the four in terms of sample size. Of the two studies focusing primarily on intellectual ability, which also considered aspects of severity, neither found evidence of a significant relationship, although duration of illness was not included as a variable. Fowler *et al.* (1986) found that scores on subscales of the WISC and the Visual Motor Integration test were not significantly correlated with numbers of days hospitalized, numbers of crises, or limitations to physical activity among 28 school-aged children with SCD, and Swift *et al.* (1989) found that the only evidence of a relationship between numbers of crises and IQ (again, using the WISC) among 21 children with sickle cell anaemia arose from one very severely affected individual.

It is difficult to be sure about why boys should have more difficulty than girls in adapting to the demands of SCD. One possibility is that the traditional activities and interests of boys of this age are less likely than those of girls to be compatible with the restrictions and limitations imposed by SCD. Factors such as overexertion, cold exposure, and changes in temperature have all been shown to be capable of precipitating sickling crises, so that boisterous physical play and strenuous outdoor activities would be more likely to lead to problems than sedentary, indoor activities. If the commonly observed gender differences in preferences for patterns of play and peer interaction (Nicholson, 1985) were assumed to apply to children with SCD, boys would be expected to be more likely than girls to risk painful crises, and to suffer restrictions and limitations to their preferred forms of play and peer interaction. Another possibility is that the child's relationships within the family might play an important role in facilitating better adjustment to SCD, and that, especially in the adolescent years, boys may tend to have more problems than girls in this area.

Family and Personality Factors

Factors relating to the family environment of children with SCD would be expected to play an important role in the coping abilities of those children, because responsibility for the management of a child's illness begins with the parents and is transferred only gradually to the child. Successful management of SCD by children would be expected to be closely related to the development of autonomous self-responsibility more generally, and might be influenced by patterns of parental protection and child care, informal education, and role models within the family. The better parents understand the condition affecting their child, the more likely they are to be able to offer useful guidance on management, for example, by pointing out links between the onset of crises and particular occasions or activities, and the less likely they would be to over-react or respond inappropriately to complications such as bed-wetting. Surveys have revealed significant levels of underinformation about SCD on the part of parents, although this factor has not to our knowledge been related directly to adjustment in children.

Some evidence is available on how more general characteristics of families such as cohesiveness, stress, and emotional expressiveness affect adjustment to SCD in children. Hurtig and Park (1989) examined adjustment to SCD in 33 adolescents aged between 12 and 17 years as a function of family styles of interaction. The results showed that, among the boys, those with fewer behavioural problems tended to be in more cohesive and expressive families, whereas in girls, those with lower levels of coping competency tended to be in more conflicting families. The authors suggested that more cohesive and expressive families would be better placed to offer emotional and physical support to adolescents with SCD, which might explain the link with reduced behavioural problems, and emphasized the need to help families develop more interactive, supportive, and organized family dynamics in order to help children and adolescents to improve their adaptation to SCD.

Moise (1986) studied 33 school-age children and adolescents with SCD (17 boys and 16 girls aged from 8 to 16) in an attempt to identify some of the individual and family factors associated with successful adjustment. Information was obtained about the children, their family environments and their progress at school from a variety of sources, using instruments which included the Norwicki–Strickland Internal–External (I–E) Scale, the Family Environment Scale, the Piers–Harris Children's Self-Concept Scale, the Stressful Life Events Checklist, the California Test of Personality (CTP), and the Child Behaviour Profile (CBP). In line with the results of previous studies, better adjusted children were in more cohesive families, and those in highly stressed families had poorer school performance.

The results also showed that better personal and social adjustment were associated with more positive self-concept, aspects of personality, and an internal locus of control. Locus of control may well be an important element of successful management, for more general theories of health psychology such as the Health Belief model (Marteau, 1989) emphasize the importance of beliefs held by people about the extent to which they are responsible for their health and are able to act effectively to improve it. King and Cross (1989) have pointed to the potential role for children with chronic illnesses to take as decision makers in the management of their conditions, and to the need to maximize children's involvement in their own care. An internal locus of control (where attributions about events focus on personal efficacy and responsibility rather than on arbitrary or environmental factors outside the individual's control) would be expected to make it more likely that an individual would perceive a condition such as SCD to be subject to their own control and thereby take a more active role in its management.

An important point to be borne in mind in relation to results showing associations between characteristics of the person and their level of successful coping is that such findings do not necessarily mean that the former is influencing the latter. For locus of control, for example, experiences of successful management could equally influence the extent to which people feel in control. This is an intrinsic limitation of all correlational studies, and prospective research, in which characteristics measured at one point in time are related to outcomes at a later date, would be needed to clarify the role of characteristics relating to personality, beliefs, and attitudes in the successful management of SCD.

Another potential complication for studies of differential adaptation to SCD is that factors relating to the individual or the family might reflect even more general differences between individuals, such as socio-economic status (Lemanek et al., 1986), or quality of available services (Kumar et al., 1976), both of which are likely to influence the extent to which individuals are able to cope with their illness. No studies of differences in coping have taken proper account of the basic circumstances in which people with SCD find themselves, aspects of which might well account for much of the variance observed in children's abilities to manage their conditions, as well as for the discrepant findings on adjustment in different samples of children with SCD.

Sickle Cell Disease and School

Katz (1980) has identified regular school attendance and participation as essential elements in children's psychosocial well-being. School provides unique opportunities for sports and leisure activities as well as for social interaction with peers, so that when things do not go well for a child at school, their personal and social development and overall quality of life may be reduced significantly. Academic achievement is also of considerable potential significance for children with SCD because of the limitations that the illness might impose on the kinds of occupations they will be able to take up as adults. People with SCD may be recommended to seek sedentary work, which does not require strenuous physical exertion. Whilst qualifications and scholastic attainment are advantages to anyone, for some people with SCD they may represent the key to the kind of working life that would allow them to manage their condition more fully.

In fact, the evidence suggests that SCD can place children at a significant disadvantage in their school careers, and parents have reported that school attendance (along with sports) was the activity most affected by pain crises (Walco and Dampier, 1990). The main problem seems to be that, like any chronic illness, SCD makes demands on the child that may, in the short term, have to take priority over education, so that time is missed from school because of infections, pain crises, disease-related problems, or the need to attend routine follow-up appointments at hospital (Shapiro et al., 1990). Fowler, Johnson, and Atkinson (1985) looked at school achievement and absenteeism in 270 chronically ill children, including some with SCD. They found that an average of more than 20 days had been missed from school during the previous academic year, the most common reasons for which were minor illnesses, the chronic health condition, and clinic visits. Children with SCD have been found to miss more time from school than their siblings (Nishiura, Whitten, and Thomas, 1982), and Shapiro et al. (1990) reported that nearly half (48 per cent) of the total of days missed from school by a sample of children with SCD were due to pain crises, although most (62 per cent) of the days missed were spent at home without attending hospital or clinic.

Absence from school would clearly be likely to affect academic achievement. Fowler et al. (1985) reported that scores on a test of school achievement were generally low among children with chronic illnesses, and Nishiura and Whitten (1980) found that one-third

67

of a sample of children with sickle cell anaemia were described by their parents as behind in school; over one-half had only fair or poor grades. Fowler *et al.* (1986) compared 28 school-aged children with SCD to a clinic sample of well children matched for age, sex, and race. They found that one-half of the SCD group had repeated a grade at school, compared with only one-fifth of the control group, and that 63 per cent, compared with 35 per cent of the controls, received special educational services.

Academic underachievement is not the only effect of enforced absence from school. Children and adolescents who are absent from school intermittently may come to feel isolated from their friends and peer groups, and may in some cases be reluctant to return. The behaviour and experiences of children when they are at school may also be influenced by the effects of their condition. Conyard *et al.* (1980) found that adjustment to school and participation in school activities was poor among children, and especially boys, with sickle cell anaemia. Many were prone to isolation, dependence, and withdrawal from relationships with peers.

As in almost every aspect of SCD, the effects of the condition on education are variable and may depend on various factors. Absence from school would be expected to be determined to a large extent by the severity of symptoms experienced, although this is probably not the only influence on school performance. In Fowler *et al.*'s (1985) study, school absence was correlated with the number of clinic visits made and with physician ratings of activity limitations, and Hurtig *et al.* (1989) have suggested that those who experience frequent and unpredictable pain crises may have the most difficulty in achieving an optimal educational performance. Performance at school probably also reflects many of the other factors that have been associated with successful adjustment more generally, and is one of the areas in which potentially negative outcomes among children with SCD could be modified by improved liaison between all those involved in the care of affected children (Walco and Dampier, 1987). Older boys seem to be particularly at risk; Hurtig (1986) reported that school performance was poorer in this group than in both older girls and younger boys.

Family factors and levels of support are also likely to influence the extent to which education is affected by illness. Moise (1986) found that children with SCD who were in highly stressed families had poorer school performance than those who were not. There is, however, no clear evidence that SCD has any direct effect on the academic potential of children. Some studies have shown that children with SCD score lower on tests of IQ than controls (Swift *et al.*, 1989), but most links with lower attainment are likely to be due to the secondary effects of absence from school, disruption to everyday routine, and lowered expectations and aspirations among affected children. One of the most important aspects of the management of chronic illness is the ability of the person concerned to maintain a reasonable level of participation and achievement in normal everyday activities, and future research should look at ways of compensating for the effects of episodic absence from school and restricted participation in school activities to enable children with SCD to make progress in education.

5

Sickle Cell Disease and the Family

Families have a massive influence on anyone who grows up in one. Parents and siblings figure prominently in the development of personality, attitudes, and abilities, and membership of a happy and functional family can be a unique asset during childhood and beyond. In this, people with SCD are no different from any others, except that the child with SCD has additional obstacles to surmount and skills to learn. In Chapter 4 we saw that factors relating to the family were among those that influence the extent to which young people with SCD cope with their condition. By providing support and assisting the development of relevant skills and attitudes, the behaviour of other family members can facilitate better coping and adjustment on the part of a child with SCD, whereas by overprotecting or setting up negative thoughts and feelings, the family can be a handicap for successful adjustment, and may constitute an obstacle in itself for the child with SCD to overcome.

As well as family influences on children with SCD, the presence of SCD in a family can affect its pattern of functioning, so that family members who are not themselves sufferers of SCD could suffer (or benefit) indirectly. Relationships between aspects of SCD and those of family functioning and adjustment can cut both ways therefore, and it may be difficult to be certain in any given case about the direction in which positive or negative influences are flowing. Relationships between individual and group factors are always complex, and those concerning the adjustment of individuals with SCD and the functioning of the families to which they belong may well be 'synergistic', in that aspects of the individual and the family may be mutually reinforcing, resulting in virtuous (or vicious) circles of interpersonal effects.

Family Factors Affecting Children with Sickle Cell Disease

The extent to which children with chronic illnesses become able to cope with their condition would be expected to be related to the quality of parental care they receive (Cappelli *et al.*, 1989). One of the most important tasks for parents with chronically ill children is to foster independence by promoting children's capacity for decision-making in the management of their condition (King and Cross, 1989). This process would be impeded by overzealous care on the part of parents, and it is a common assumption that chronically ill children are overindulged and overprotected by their parents. In fact, the evidence suggests that although over-protection is generally counterproductive, it is not actually more prevalent among the parents of chronically ill children. In a study of parental care and overprotection among children with cystic fibrosis and healthy controls, Cappelli *et al.* (1989) found no signifi-cant differences in parental behaviour between the groups, but poorer psychosocial functioning among the children was associ-ated with overprotection in those with cystic fibrosis, and with lack of parental care in the controls.

Recent evidence from interviews with families suggests that parents do not treat children with SCD differently to their other children (Midence, Davies, and Fuggle, 1992a), and that children with SCD do not perceive their condition to have had a negative effect on their relationship with their parents (Midence *et al.* 1992b). In some cases, SCD had a positive effect on family func-tioning and enabled families to become closer and more suppor-tive. Care and protection is usually welcome and appropriate during painful crises, but children with SCD may experience helplessness and dependency if their parents treat them as if they were continuously ill, so that it is between crises that the parents are at greatest risk of overprotecting children with SCD (LePon-tois, 1986).

Irrespective of whether children with SCD are treated diffe-rently or overprotected by their parents, their adjustment would be expected to be influenced by the general quality of their family environment. Family dynamics can influence the course of chronic illnesses in an individual, and increased cohesion in families has been shown to facilitate problem-solving skills and more open expression of emotion (Minuchin *et al.* 1975). In a study of the families of children with diabetes, Marteau, Bloch, and Baum

72

(1987) found that better control of blood glucose was related to factors such as cohesion, expressiveness, lack of conflict, and the mother's satisfaction with her marriage.

In this respect the results of studies of families affected by SCD are broadly in line with those of other chronic illnesses. Moise (1986) found that among school-aged children with SCD, those who were better adjusted were more likely to come from more cohesive families, and those with poorer school performances were more likely to come from highly stressed families. Hurtig and Park (1989) looked at coping in adolescents with SCD as a function of family styles, and found that cohesive and expressive families were associated with fewer behavioural problems among the boys and greater coping competency among the girls. Similar results were found by Evans, Burlew, and Oler (1988). Hurtig and Park suggested that more interactive, supportive, and organized family dynamics would help young people adapt to SCD, and that emotional as well as physical support, allowing open and direct expression of feelings, would contribute to the reduction of behavioural problems. Other authors (Kumar *et al.*, 1976; Lemanek *et al.*, 1986) have suggested that, where good family support and effective health care are available, the psychosocial adjustment of children with SCD should not suffer, although guidance and reassurance are important to promote confidence and positive self-concept.

The importance of open, frank discussion of feelings and concerns between parents and children with SCD has been considered by Whitten and Fischoff (1974). They suggested that a child's difficulty in expressing fear or other feelings may be due to cues picked up from the parents indicating that such topics are taboo. Parents could be encouraged to deal with their own fears in order to facilitate open communication between themselves and their children and to clarify any misconceptions and myths about the illness that the family may have.

The quality of a child's family environment will depend on various factors, including the personalities and attitudes of the individuals concerned and their level of knowledge about SCD. It may also be related to factors outside the family's direct control, such as conditions of housing and employment, income, and recreational opportunities. Lemanek *et al.* (1986), for example, suggested that the behavioural problems they found among children with SCD and healthy controls could be attributed to social and economic factors associated with poverty and minority status, rather than to SCD or more specific family characteristics.

Effects of Sickle Cell Disease on the Family

A sizeable literature exists on the way that chronic illness gene-rally can affect families and the lifestyles of family members (Grath, 1977; Weiss, 1981; Sargent, 1983; Turk and Kerns, 1985). By contrast, very little is known about the family-related implica-tions of SCD, for researchers have almost completely ignored the presence of chronic illness (not just SCD) in black families. Differ-ences in family structure and dynamics, religion, formal and informal networks, available community support and resources, and experiences of racism mean that findings cannot be general-ized from one ethnic population to another. Some of the social and cultural features associated with black families might be expected to assist them in accommodating chronic illness whereas others may militate against successful adaptation, but until more is known (or acknowledged) about the way that ethnic factors affect family adaptation to chronic illness, the scope for improvements in the provision of effective psychological and social support servi-ces to ethnic minorities will be significantly restricted. A further limitation of the literature is that most of the studies have been based on the traditional two-parent model of the family, so that the effects of chronic illness in one-parent families have been neglected (Shapiro and Wallace, 1987).

Families of children with chronic illnesses have sometimes been considered to be different in some way from those of healthy children (Pless, 1985; Spaulding and Morgan, 1986). In psycho-social terms, however, the evidence suggests that they do not differ significantly (Hobbs, Perrin and Ireys, 1985), and a recent epide-miological study (Cadman et al., 1991) found that the families of children with chronic illness or physical disability did not show any marked indications of maladjustment compared with those of healthy children. Considerable variation would be expected between families however, with some being affected far more than others by the presence of a member with a chronic illness. Predict-ably, the same types of family factors, such as communication and quality of interaction, which have been associated with more positive outcomes among affected children have also been shown to be related to the psychological well being of the family as a whole (Minuchin, Rosman and Baker, 1978; Moos, 1984).

Parents

Information and Knowledge

Information is a critical factor in parents' ability to cope effectively with SCD in the family. Detailed medical understanding is not necessary, but basic knowledge about how to prevent crises and what to do during painful episodes is a prerequisite for proper management of the condition (Smith, 1980; Midence and Shand, 1992). In spite of this, there is evidence that parents are often underinformed about SCD.

Major problems could be created where no one attempts to inform patients and parents about the condition and how they might learn to cope with it. Anionwu and Beattie (1981) reported that many parents complained that they had been given little or no information about the condition. As a result, they lacked the skills to prevent or cope with some of the many problems that arose, and this could create additional feelings of fear, helplessness, and depression.

Health professionals may be confused about exactly whose role it is to impart information, and there may be a fear of exaggerating the dangers and alarming parents unnecessarily (Whitten and Fischoff, 1974), but there would seem to be a strong case for beginning sensitive health education as early as possible. Parents have reported a lack of awareness and information even before the birth of a child with SCD, and at the time of diagnosis, when mothers reported not fully understanding what they were told (Midence et al., 1992a).

The affected child is not the only loser when parents know too little about a condition like SCD, although it may certainly be exposed to unnecessary suffering. Parents have reported feeling frustration, anxiety, guilt, overprotective impulses, depression, and hopelessness during their children's pain crises (Whitten and Fischoff, 1974; Anionwu and Beattie, 1981; Midence et al., 1992b). Feelings like this may reflect underlying psychosocial difficulties and inability to cope effectively with SCD (Graham et al. 1982), but even where parents are in fact doing everything necessary and possible, ignorance about the condition could only exacerbate any fears and anxieties parents may have, and may make family conflicts and disagreements more difficult to resolve.

75

Strain on the Parental Relationship

There is no large-scale, reliable evidence available on rates of divorce and relationship problems associated with the presence of a child with SCD in the family, but there is good reason to suppose that considerable strain could be placed on the parents' relationship. In chronic illness generally, marital conflict and strain is more common among affected families (Burr, 1985; Johnson, 1985; Perrin and MacLean, 1988), although rates of divorce are not higher than among comparable families without chronic illness (Sabbeth and Leventhal, 1984). Strain and conflict between parents is not inevitable though; Ferrari (1984) found that some parents reported improvements in the quality of their relationship and the closeness of the family as a result of having a chronically ill child in the family.

In Midence *et al.*'s (1992a) interview study of mothers of children with SCD, several mothers were bringing up children alone, although in only one case out of ten was the relationship between parents considered to have been ended as a direct result of SCD. In a study conducted in Nigeria, Bamisaiye, Bakare, and Olatawura (1974) found that over 63 per cent of fathers and 93 per cent of mothers felt that SCD in their children had made the marriage an unhappy one.

Among chronic illnesses, inherited conditions like SCD have perhaps the greatest potential for causing difficulties in the parents' relationship. If parents are aware in advance of the risk to their children (because both are sufferers themselves, or carry the trait), they will have difficult decisions to make about whether to have children and whether to terminate a pregnancy when prenatal diagnosis indicates SCD. Where SCD presents itself unexpectedly, parents may blame themselves or one another for passing the condition to their children, and the birth of a child with SCD or the results of a screening programme for the trait occasionally brings to light facts about the true paternity of the child, which would otherwise not have arisen.

This is because the genetic status of the father in relation to sickle cell can be inferred from that of the mother and the child. For example, if a child is born with the full form (SS) of SCD, and the mother's partner is not a carrier of the sickle cell gene (AS), then he can only be the biological father if a spontaneous genetic mutation has occurred. Alternatively, if the child is found to be AS (trait) by a routine screen and the mother is not, then the biological father very probably is, and the husband or partner's paternity will be in serious doubt if he does not carry the trait. This makes screening and testing for sickle cell disease a highly sensitive issue in a few cases, in which most of the burden will fall on the mother to decide whether to be tested for the trait, and how to cope with the issues raised by non-paternity.

Mothers

In general, and for various reasons, mothers rather than fathers bear the main burden of caring for children with chronic illnesses. In diabetes and cystic fibrosis, for example, mothers have been found to be more knowledgeable than fathers about the child's illness (Johnson *et al.* 1982; Nolan *et al.*, 1986), and Eiser (1990a) has suggested that findings like these reflect differential involvement in the day-to-day care of the child with chronic illness.

Many studies of mothers with chronically ill children have shown that the child's condition affects the mother's mental and physical health. Such women appear to have poorer mental health than either fathers of chronically ill children or mothers of healthy children. Jessop, Riessman, and Stein (1988) studied the mothers of 209 children with different chronic illnesses, and found that poor mental health among mothers was related to their perception of the severity of their child's condition. The absence of emotional support, the presence of other stressful factors, the impact of the condition on the family, and the women's physical health were also predictive of psychiatric symptoms among mothers.

Mothers of children with SCD would appear to be at similar risk. A survey of affected families in Newham, London, found that 88 per cent of the mothers interviewed felt that their lives had been affected by SCD (Black and Laws, 1986). The most commonly reported problems were worry and the need to take time off work. Many mothers either did not work or had to work part-time or at night in order to look after their children. Midence *et al.* (1992a) also found that mothers reported disruption of their work and social life because of the need to be available at all times and constant worry about the child's next pain crisis. Other feelings reported by mothers of children with SCD include being emotionally overwhelmed (Anionwu and Beattie, 1981), stress due to the burden of coping (Sellers, 1975), hopelessness and frustration during pain crises (Abrams, 1987), and the need for social support (Slaughter and Anderson, 1985).

Fathers

The roles played by fathers in families of children with SCD, and chronic illness more generally, have not so far been widely investigated, probably because the assumption has been that the responsibility for the care of such children falls predominantly on mothers (King, 1981). The results of a survey of the parents of children with SCD in Nigeria were broadly in line with this assumption; only 33 per cent of fathers, compared with 80 per cent of mothers, reported that their working lives had been affected by their child's condition (Bamisaiye *et al.*, 1974).

Even where the father plays only a subsidiary role in the direct care for children, he is likely to have a distinct influence on the development of personality, values, and attitudes of children. This aspect of parenting is only beginning to be investigated within developmental psychology generally. In children with chronic illnesses, the influence of fathers may be of critical importance as children learn strategies for coping and achieving independence. It would be expected to be particularly important for male children, given that the father is potentially an important role model, and that the young boy with a chronic illness may be casting about for suitable models in an effort to adapt to the constraints of his illness.

Research is needed on the ways that fathers respond to the presence of SCD in the family, how they are affected psychologically, how they treat children with SCD compared with healthy siblings, how their responses to children with SCD differ from those of the mother, and what contribution they make to overall patterns of family functioning and interaction in families affected by SCD.

The role of partners or fathers in families of children with SCD, and chronic illness more generally, is therefore an area that needs to be explored in much more detail. Fathers and male partners would need to be incorporated in any model which attempted to explain the mechanisms involved in the coping and management of SCD in families.

Siblings

Some research has suggested that behavioural and emotional problems in healthy children are more common among those who have a chronically ill brother or sister (Lavigne and Ryan, 1979; Tritt, 1984); the evidence is not clear-cut, however. Cadman (1987) found that the siblings of chronically ill children generally enjoyed good mental health and social well-being. Breslau, Weitzman, and Messenger (1981) conducted a comprehensive study of 239 families of disabled children, showing that siblings did not differ from controls in terms of psychological impairment and lack of parental attention. One explanation for the discrepant findings in this area may be that healthy siblings of sick children are at increased risk of maladjustment only where other factors are also present (Drotar and Crawford, 1985). Specific aspects of the condition, rather than simply the presence of illness, may also influence the extent to which siblings are affected (Ferrari, 1984).

Chronic illness in the family may also affect siblings in more positive ways, by making them more compassionate, understanding, or sensitive (Grossman, 1972). Ferrari (1984) found that, according to their teachers, siblings of children with diabetes displayed the most prosocial behaviour towards other children at school, and that siblings of disabled children were given the highest ratings for social competence. Many of the parents also reported that siblings were more compassionate and understanding as a result of having a chronically ill brother or sister.

The way in which children might respond to chronic illness in a brother or sister is clearly complex, and would be expected to reflect factors such as the nature of the illness and the overall pattern of relationships within the family, especially the parents' treatment of both sick and healthy siblings. In the absence of reliable evidence it is impossible to generalize about how siblings might respond to SCD, and any studies in this area would also need to take into account features of parental and sibling interaction, which may be characteristic of black families. They would also need to consider how family responses to SCD might be affected by the presence of more than one person with SCD in the family, whether a parent and a child, both parents, or more than one child were affected.

The only direct evidence on the question of sibling effects in SCD was inconclusive. Abrams (1987) assessed the 'self-concepts' of 20 children with SCD but no siblings, 20 children with SCD and healthy siblings, and 20 healthy control siblings, using the Piers–Harris Children's Self-concept Scale. There were no significant differences between the three groups, although most of the children generally had low scores on the positive self-concept scale.

79

The Financial Cost of Sickle Cell Disease

Chronic illness is almost always a financial liability. In many cases the additional expense cannot easily be absorbed by the family budget, and may be a significant factor in the overall impact of the illness on the family (Stein and Riessman, 1980). Surveys have shown that around 60 per cent of parents with chronically ill children had experienced financial problems through the costs of dietary requirements, living arrangements, travelling expenses, time missed from work, clothing, and heating (Satterwhite, 1978). Higher levels of financial stress have also been found among families with physically disabled children compared with controls (Singhi et al., 1990).

Many researchers have documented the financial difficulties experienced by families because of SCD (Nishiura and Whitten, 1980; Collins, 1986; Midence et al., 1992a). Managing crises requires dressing warmly, drinking fluids frequently, and having a telephone available at a very minimum, and may extend to keeping the heating on all year round. Family income may also be affected by the need for parents to be at home or at hospital from time to time. In many cases these costs have to be borne by low income or single parent families living in disadvantaged areas and struggling in any case to make ends meet.

Financial restrictions have various important social and psychological implications. Opportunities for recreation and social interaction may be limited (Kessler and Cleary, 1980) and this can influence personal development and quality of life, almost invariably for the worse. In children with asthma, higher levels of maladjustment were found among those from families in poorer accommodation or where mothers had no access to a car (Anderson et al., 1983). Pless et al. (1989) found that, among a large sample of adolescents and adults who had suffered from various chronic illnesses during their childhood, those from families of lower socio-economic groups tended to be in significantly worse social and psychological circumstances. Even at 36 years of age, they were worse off in terms of opportunities and basic social support. It comes as no surprise, therefore, to find that sociodemographic factors are among those most closely associated with outcomes among children with SCD. Higher income levels or better financial support may enable families to manage SCD better, to compensate for some of the limitations it imposes, and to give children the opportunity to participate in a wider range of activities outside the home, all of which are important factors in psychological adjustment and well-being.

Support for the Family

External support for the family may come from organized professional bodies in the voluntary or statutory sector, or from informal networks and contacts within the community, including the extended family, friends, and neighbours. It can take the form of financial assistance and specific services relating to childcare, housing or health, or less tangible services such as sympathy, advice, or listening skills. The importance of social support of all types in promoting physical and psychological health is widely recognized (Cohen and Syme, 1985), and is of particular relevance where families who are already in difficult circumstances have to cope with the additional demands imposed by chronic illnesses (Minuchin et al., 1978; Satariano and Syme, 1981).

Broadhead et al. (1983) have suggested that helping to avoid stressful and difficult situations and providing some measure of protection when such situations are encountered are among the most important ways in which families benefit psychologically from external support. Exposure to stressful situations has been found to be related to maladjustment in families affected by chronic illness (Varni and Wallander, 1988), and Kazak (1987) has shown how professional support from medical, educational, and social services can help to reduce the experience of stress. Stressful events in families with SCD have also been reduced by the availability of greater social support (Leavell and Ford, 1983).

Informal networks of family support are features of the black community, with high levels of co-operation and sharing contributing to a distinct cultural tradition (Aschenbrenner, 1975). This type of support has various aspects. McAdoo (1978) found that child care was the most important component of the family exchange system, and Martin and Martin (1978) have described the importance of emotional support in troubled times, including the knowledge that someone was available who cared and who could be turned to in times of crisis.

It is perhaps not surprising that social support has been described by families of children with SCD as the single most important factor associated with successful coping (Smith, 1980; Midence et al., 1992a). Lester (1986) interviewed 33 parents of children with sickle cell anaemia to identify the most important forms of social support. Simple things such as companionship, empathy, and verbal support during pain crises were described by parents as the most helpful.

The advantages to parents of becoming involved with other parents of children with SCD in self-help groups or SCD societies in the community has been emphasized by Flanagan (1980). Groups like this can help to reduce tension in the home environment by exploring the feelings, attitudes, and fears of children and adults, and by providing a forum for the discussion of feelings, for example, the fear of death, which are often experienced but rarely expressed in one-to-one talk between parent and child. Even very young children can be included in discussions about the disease and its management, beginning with simple explanations of the implications of the condition and gradually involving them in the management of the condition as they grow older.

One of the most significant features of this area is the ability of many families to cope remarkably well with SCD. Part of the reason for this may be the co-operative and supportive culture of the black community. There is, however, an urgent need to examine and improve the delivery of formal services to families, including basic provision and access, and more complex social and psychological services, in order to improve the circumstances of families who are coping less well than they could. To do this, the unique heritage of black families with their cultural and subcultural differences need to be better understood and addressed more directly. The social and psychological processes related to family dynamics, such as religion, family structure, racial discrimination, and the use of formal and informal networks by the black community, need to be investigated if better psychological and social services are to be offered to these families.

6

Sickle Cell Disease in Adulthood

At one time, very few people with the full form of SCD survived to adulthood. Greater medical understanding and more effective measures against infections and other complications mean that people with SCD are now living longer. Most reach adulthood (Leikin *et al.*, 1989), and some live to their 50s, 60s, and 70s (Brozovic and Davies, 1987; Gray *et al.*, 1991). Although the clinical presentation of SCD changes to some extent over the lifespan, with different complications arising at different ages, the most important features of the condition remain the same, namely unpredictable painful episodes and restrictions and limitations to activities and lifestyle. The severity of the condition and the extent to which people are affected also remain highly variable, although the areas of life in which problems might arise, and the factors that influence better coping and adaptation would be expected to differ from those that are relevant to adjustment in children.

Various aspects of adult life have potentially important consequences for adaptation to SCD, some of which might be expected to act for the better and others for the worse. As young people reach adulthood they are usually protected less by family and caring institutions, and must take greater responsibility for the management of their condition. They may also be exposed to popular misconceptions and prejudices about SCD to a far greater extent, and may face new and difficult challenges in the workplace and social life.

There have been fewer studies of adults with SCD than of children, although the main areas of investigation, namely psychological adjustment, coping strategies, and effects on lifestyle have been similar, with more emphasis on active coping and adjustment in adults. A regrettable gap in the picture presented by research on this topic is that of the transition from childhood to adulthood, for there have been no longitudinal studies of adjustment over the lifespan. This means that it is not possible to make reliable assessments of the ways and the extent to which adjustment later in life is influenced by events and experiences in childhood, or to draw conclusions about whether, and how, the apparently increased difficulty experienced by older children is reflected in the adjustment of adults.

In this chapter we first consider aspects of the clinical presentation of SCD that are likely to change with age, or are likely to affect adults in different ways from children, including patterns of pain and complications such as leg ulcers and priapism. We go on to look at psychological adjustment among adults with SCD in terms of psychiatric disturbance and coping strategies. Finally, we consider the social and economic implications for adults with SCD, including socializing, parenting, and working.

Clinical Presentation

Pain

The main differences between SCD pain in childhood and in adulthood is that in adults the pain is more central in distribution and more severe, with longer hospital stays. Adults will usually also have had more experience of painful crises. There is no reason to believe that increasing age makes sickling either more or less likely in physiological terms, but behavioural factors in relation to the avoidance and management of SCD pain might be expected to reduce the impact of painful crises as the affected person grows older. Adults would have had greater opportunity for learning about the kinds of activities and situations that had preceded crises in the past, and about the most effective ways to respond to the onset of pain. On the other hand, repeated experience of pain might have a cumulative emotional effect, reducing the individual's capacity to maintain psychological well being by undermining their self-confidence and chipping away at their feelings of control. The subjective experience of pain is distressing at any age, and adults may have just as much difficulty as children in coming to terms with both the effects and the unpredictability of pain crises (Daniels, 1990).

The main way in which adults would be expected to gain from their experience with SCD pain is that they would know more about the kinds of activities and situations that were likely to precipitate crises. However, their scope for avoiding such circumstances may itself be limited by factors outside their direct control, such as the type of work and housing they are able to obtain, and benefits obtained in this way could be regarded simply as trade-offs made by the individual between forgoing or curtailing activities and risking an episode of pain. However, choices of this kind must be made by anyone with SCD, and experience would be expected to increase an individual's ability to find the balance that improves their quality of life. As the person with SCD grows older, they would also be expected to become more skilled in the management of pain, and they should be better placed than a child to respond promptly and appropriately at the onset of a painful episode.

However, any overall benefits in adjustment obtained through increased experience are likely to be marginal by comparison with the effects of differences between people of any age in terms of the extent of their pain problem and of their coping resources. A significant minority (around one-fifth) of adults with SCD experience frequent crises for which hospitalization is required (Williams, Earles, and Pack, 1983), whereas others are symptom-free for long periods. In a study of acute admissions in SCD, Brozovic *et al.* (1987) found that 6 per cent of patients accounted for over 40 per cent of all admissions. Ruchnagel (1974), for example, has commented that: 'increasingly, individuals are encountered with apparent SCD who seldom experience episodes of severe pains ... or who live to the 6th or 7th decade'.

The majority of adults with SCD experience fewer but more severe painful crises than in childhood. Most should be able to expect a reasonable life expectancy and extended periods of good health, but their quality of life and level of adjustment will also be influenced by the extent to which they have been able to benefit from past experience in the management of crises. This would depend upon the level and quality of service available to them at present and in the past, the relationship they have with their doctors, and their attitudes and beliefs in relation to their condition and their ability to manage it.

Other Problems

Some of the medical complications associated with SCD are much more common in later life, or affect adults to a much greater extent than children. These include leg ulcers, priapism, and aspects of SCD relevant to contraception and childbirth.

Leg Ulcers

Leg ulcerations are one of the less well understood complications of SCD, but affect large numbers of older children and adults with sickle cell anaemia in the tropics (Chernoff, Shapleigh, and Moore, 1954), and account for a good deal of pain, absence from work, decreased activity, and embarrassment. Leg ulcers are much less common in the UK and the USA, and SC individuals are less severely affected (Koshy et al., 1989). Leg ulcers are probably caused when minor cuts and abrasions fail to heal normally because of poor blood flow in the affected area. Treatment consists of careful cleaning and dressing over a period of weeks or months, but there remains a high risk of recurrence (Noel, 1983).

Some of the social and psychological consequences of leg ulcers were examined by Alleyne, Wint, and Serjeant (1977), who compared 36 affected people over the age of 17 with 35 people who also had sickle cell anaemia but no history of leg ulceration. Failure to accept SCD was twice as common among those with leg ulcers (29 per cent compared with 14 per cent), and 16 people reported that they had left school early because of their leg ulcers. Ulcers are one of the few visible and unsightly complications of SCD, so that the potential for stigmatization in those affected could be increased by embarrassment and inhibition about dress, social activities, and the possible responses of others.

Priapism

Priapism is a persistent and abnormal erection of the penis accompanied by pain, tenderness, and swelling. It may or may not be associated with sexual arousal, but is not relieved by sexual activity (Hauri, Spycher, and Bruhlmann, 1983). Sickling causes priapism by occluding the circulatory spaces and small blood vessels of the penis and obstructing the drainage of blood from the corpora cavernosa (Schmidt and Flocks, 1971). Around one-quarter of all reported cases of priapism occur in men with SCD (Ihekwaba, 1980), of whom 10 to 15 per cent suffer what is among the least investigated complications of SCD (Franklin, 1990). It does not usually present before the age of five, and is most common in men who are sexually active. Episodes can last for days or weeks and can be among the most frightening and disturbing complications of SCD, with potentially significant physical and psychological effects. The most important of these obviously relate to the sexual lives of affected men and their partners. Episodes of priapism can begin with sexual intercourse, so that sexual enjoyment might be impaired by anxiety about future attacks, and prolonged episodes of priapism can lead to partial or complete impotence. Self-confidence and self-esteem may be reduced because those affected feel they are not able to perform adequately, or feel that their masculinity has been compromised.

In extreme cases, exchange blood transfusion and even surgery may be needed to drain blood from the penis, which relieves engorgement and pain. Both protracted priapism and surgery for its relief carry a risk of impotence and chordee (angulation of the penis). More conservative therapies include hydration, analgesia, hot or cold packs, irrigation, and a variety of other measures (Hamre et al., 1991). It is important that priapism is not neglected, for successful outcomes have been associated with early presentation and therapeutic intervention (Bertram, Webster, and Carson, 1985), but embarrassment and awkwardness on the part of both patients and medical staff may mean that the problem does not get effective attention early enough.

Fertility, Contraception, and Childbirth

Women, and, to a lesser extent, men with SCD are potentially vulnerable to complications related to fertility, contraception, and childbirth. In males, lower semen volume, sperm counts, and sperm motility have all been observed (Davies, 1988b), for reasons that are not yet clear, but that must relate to sickling in the testes.

There is no evidence that female fertility is affected by SCD, but pregnancy is potentially problematic. Early pregnancy is generally not complicated, but difficulties arise more frequently during the final third of the term and during labour, including more frequent severe pain crises. Pregnancy and labour put added strains on the body, and problems may arise with the use of anaesthetics (Tuck, 1982). Other possible complications include preterm labour, liver dysfunction, low iron levels, urinary tract infection, toxaemia, pre-eclampsia, avascular necrosis, and retinopathy.

The risk of complication and morbidity also apply to the fetus of a pregnant woman with SCD, which may be affected by poor fetal growth (caused by maternal anaemia), prematurity, and low birth weight. Maternal SCD is also associated with increased rates of stillbirth, spontaneous abortion, and miscarriage.

Contraception

People who may be making difficult decisions about family planning need access to the best available contraceptive services and advice. Choices about contraceptive methods may be more difficult for women with SCD because the coil may cause complications and the pill can be dangerous (Serjeant, 1983) and is not recommended in all countries. This might be a loss for women who would prefer to be on the pill in order to control menstrual difficulties, which are sometimes associated with SCD. Some women find that their periods tend to set off painful sickling crises. There would appear to be no additional risk associated with the low-dose combined pill or progesterone-only preparations though, and depoprovera (an injectable progesterone that acts over a period of months) may actually inhibit sickling (De Ceular *et al.*, 1982), although its safety has not been proven for women with or without SCD. Barrier methods (the condom and the diaphragm) can be used without any risk of complications, and sterilization or vasectomy are also low-risk options that may be suitable for couples in stable relationships.

A woman with SCD may have her contraceptive options limited or complicated, and supportive co-operation by her partner should not be taken for granted. Black and Laws (1986) reported comments made by many of the women they interviewed about their husbands' and boyfriends' resistance to using condoms. Vasectomy of the male is an option only for certain women, and for many the options are the diaphragm, the low-dose combined pill, the progesterone pill, or sterilization, which may be viewed more favourably by some doctors than patients. Black and Laws (1986, p. 203) commented:

> Five out of the seven women in our sample who have children had been sterilized. We are not confident that all of these women had given informed consent to these operations, many of which were done immediately after childbirth.

It is very important that women with SCD be given the correct advice and information about contraception, but less knowledgeable medical staff may overestimate the dangers of pregnancy. Many of the women interviewed by Black and Laws reported that they had been warned against dire consequences and told never to become pregnant. Problems may be created because women go to different agencies for different aspects of health care. Many GPs or doctors in family planning clinics know little about SCD, whereas haematologists and SCD counsellors may not cover contraception adequately. Family planning is a good example of the need for closer integration of services for people with SCD.

Pregnancy
Some women with SCD experience straightforward pregnancies and give birth to healthy babies. Others may encounter serious complications related to SCD, and medical monitoring and support should be available during this critical time. Antenatal diagnosis for SCD should be available for all at-risk couples. This provides the option of termination, although all of the available methods for testing the haemoglobin type of the fetus carry some risk of miscarriage. Amniocentesis can be conducted from 14 to 16 weeks from conception, chorionic villus sampling (CVS) can be performed between the tenth and sixteenth weeks of gestation, and fetal blood sampling from 18 to 22 weeks; the fetal tissue is usually analysed using DNA techniques.

Murray *et al.* (1980) have pointed out some of the issues that arise in relation to the provision of prenatal diagnostic techniques for people of ethnic and racial minorities. The perspectives and attitudes of minority groups may differ from those of the majority in ways that are influenced by cultural, linguistic, social, educational, and economic factors, along with differential access to diagnostic and therapeutic services, all of which may contribute to a generalized suspicion and fear of institutional manipulation and control. However, antenatal diagnosis during the first trimester of pregnancy is overwhelmingly popular among women with SCD (Jones *et al.*, 1988), and there is evidence that early diagnosis and regular follow-up reduces morbidity amongst those who receive support, so that prompt diagnosis of SCD can itself play a role in improving the prognosis of those affected.

Attitudes to abortion vary and there are various issues, both ethical and practical, that need to be taken into account when considering the termination of a pregnancy in which SCD is indicated (Anionwu, 1983). What makes the decision most difficult is that the course and severity of SCD is at present almost impossible to predict. Our view is that SCD should not be regarded *in itself* as grounds for terminating a pregnancy, given the potential for effective support and the fact that increasing numbers of affected people lead long lives and go on to become parents themselves. However, any decision about terminating a pregnancy should rest finally with the mother, whose circumstances and perceptions of the various options might lead to choices that others would not agree with. The role of a nurse counsellor is to provide support regardless of the decision.

Psychological Adjustment

Adults with SCD have been compared less frequently than children to people without SCD or with other chronic illnesses. The results of such studies, however, are generally more consistent than those of children, and seem to indicate a risk of psychological disturbance associated with SCD. Depression appears to be a common problem and has been linked to aspects of the condition, the circumstances of the person, and their ability to cope, at least some of which could be changed to reduce the risk of disturbance.

Thompson et al. (1992) looked at 109 adults with SCD in North Carolina, using a checklist of behavioural and emotional symptoms. Over half (56 per cent) met criteria for poor adjustment of one kind or another, with 40 per cent showing signs of depression and 32 per cent signs of anxiety. Two studies have found higher levels of disturbance among people with SCD than those with diabetes. Damlouji et al. (1982) compared adults with SCD to adults with diabetes of the same race and socio-economic group. They found that 63 per cent of those with SCD showed signs of psychiatric morbidity, compared with 50 per cent of those with diabetes. Charache, Lubin, and Reid (1984) found higher levels of depression, but also of disability, in 30 people with SCD than in a comparison group of people with diabetes.

Disturbances of mood and emotion would perhaps be expected in a condition associated with episodic pain and there is a strong prima facie case for a link between painful episodes and depression (Morin and Waring, 1981), but it is by no means clear how the link operates in every case. Given that chronic undertreated pain generally has been shown to be capable of inducing feelings and behaviour characteristic of clinical depression (see Chapter 3), frequency or severity of pain would be expected to play an important causal role, but there is also evidence that depression, usually in response to adverse circumstances, can precede pain crises. Nadel and Portadin (1977), for example, found that of 22 people with SCD aged between 16 and 35 years, half reported that the onset of painful crises was preceded by severe depressive effects such as helplessness and hopelessness, which were in response to different types of loss, mainly unemployment. Retrospective studies like this should perhaps be treated with caution to the extent that scope might exist for subjects (or investigators) to make attributions with hindsight about the causes of pain crises, but it seems possible that depression or affective disorders could influence the incidence of pain crises by disrupting coping behaviour.

However, clinical depressive illness is characterized by mood states and behaviours that persist over changes in circumstances, so that findings of depressive symptoms as a precursor or as a consequence of pain crises is not convincing evidence of a risk of mental illness for SCD *per se*. There is also evidence that many of the apparently 'psychopathological' problems observed in SCD do not in fact require psychiatric care, but can be countered effectively by more general improvements in the advice, support and information provided to the individual. Leavell and Ford (1983), for example, looked at adjustment in eight male and eight female adults, aged between 19 and 53, with SCD. 'Adjustment' ranged from 'normal' to 'severe psychopathology', but symptomatic expression of SCD was associated with life stress and was reduced by increasing the availability of social support. Collins (1986), who looked at psychosocial problems in a sample of 386 adults with SCD aged between 19 and 50, found that the most common were treatment compliance difficulties, family or relationship problems, poor relationships with health professionals, mood disturbance, and financial difficulties. Many of these were addressed successfully by providing better counselling or emotional support, or by improving the liaison between medical, social service, and counselling staff. Others responded to simple behavioural methods such as instruction, reinforcement, or the use of strategies to monitor specific problems.

Behavioural or psychological interventions of this nature could be said to address problems in 'adjustment' more directly, without looking for causes in the person's medical condition or physical and social environment. Neither do they assume an underlying psychological abnormality, but instead consider problems in adjustment (firstly at least) as responses to circumstances that would be expected to conform with what is already known about health psychology and human behaviour generally.

Cognitive Factors

Relationships between phenomena in the external, physiological, and psychological worlds are never straightforward, and it is likely that factors of all three types have the potential to influence one another in various ways and to different extents, so that no single mechanism could account fully for the links between SCD and relatively poor adjustment. Direct causation of depression by pain would not explain why adjustment is not more closely linked with factors such as frequency or severity of pain. On the other hand, explanations of depression in terms only of environmental factors would not account for the findings of a higher incidence of psychopathology in people with SCD than in matched controls. Any relationships between illness, adjustment, and environment would be mediated by factors such as perception, attitudes, knowledge, behavioural styles, and use of coping strategies, and cognitive factors of this kind may be much better predictors of overall adjustment than either illness or environmental factors.

Gil *et al.* (1989) looked at the relationship between coping styles and adjustment to SCD pain in 79 adults, using structured interviews and self-report questionnaires to assess coping strategies used and distress experienced. The results showed that use of strategies predicted a significant proportion of the variance in adjustment to SCD. People whose coping styles were characterized by 'negative thinking' and 'passive adherence' reported more severe pain crises, more frequent hospitalizations, higher levels of distress, and lower levels of activity during crises, whereas those who reported more 'coping attempts' also reported more activity during crises.

Although studies like this do not rule out the possibility that the cognitive factors under investigation were themselves just part of the responses to distress, it seems highly likely that perceptions, beliefs, and coping styles influence the extent to which people with SCD are able to make effective adjustments to their condition. Locus of control (see chapter 4) has not been investigated in adults with SCD, but results like those of Gil *et al.* (1989) suggest that those who believe strongly that they have the ability to influence their health would be less likely, other things being equal, to experience problems in psychological adjustment. Many personal accounts, such as Daniels (1990), emphasize the importance of learning to live with SCD at a personal level in order to reduce its impact on quality of life. Phillips (1976), for example, pointed out:

One has to learn to accept such a condition ... learning how to accept an affliction of any kind is not an easy thing ... But I am more certain that the more facts we have available, the better we are able to move decisively. This kind of action can give a feeling of mastery. Attaining such mastery decreases our anxieties and increases our sense of confidence and security.

The Stress Perspective

A very broad conceptual framework in which illness, environment, and cognitive factors can all be accommodated in a rudimentary way is that of stress. Looking at adaptation to chronic illness from a stress perspective involves making a functional analysis of the person and their environment as a system of interrelated parts, which must maintain certain conditions if it is not to break down. Stress is caused by inflexibility in the relations between parts when the system is operating uncomfortably close to its limits. When the sum of the demands on the system, such as maintaining an income and a social life, keeping painful episodes to a minimum, and avoiding depressive reactions to SCD, are only barely matched by the sum of the economic, social, medical and psychological resources available to the system, there is less margin for error, and the person experiences stress, which could express itself in various, and variously predictable, ways. More stable factors may influence individual susceptibility to stress, but temporary or situational factors would determine the form and the timing of expressions of stress. Some of these may meet standard criteria for psychopathology, but many probably do not.

Thompson *et al.* (1992) looked at psychological adjustment in 109 adults with SCD in North Carolina, in relation to aspects of stress and coping. Adjustment, as indicated by a checklist of psychological symptoms, was not associated with factors such as type of illness, or measures of severity (numbers of complications and frequency of pain), but was predicted by measures of perceived stress associated with daily hassles. The authors suggested that stress management training would be a useful aid to coping for people with SCD.

Is Age a Factor?

It is interesting to note the contrasting patterns of results obtained in studies of psychological disturbance among children and adults

93

with SCD. The findings of adult studies are much more consistent than those of children, and seem to indicate a risk of psychopathology among people with SCD. Several factors might contribute to this. First, the adult studies have generally used a narrower range of constructs, focusing principally on psychopathological criteria, whereas the studies of children covered aspects of personality, intellectual functioning, behavioural observations, and other measures of adjustment. This would make consistent findings more likely among the studies of adults. However, part of the reason for the choice of measures for the studies of children was probably that psychopathology is problematic to identify reliably in children, and occurs more frequently in early adulthood. It is possible that a wider range of less predictable signs and symptoms in early life are markers for better defined syndromes in adulthood, and that chronic pain and limitations to activities, combined with less effective management – which may itself be related to behavioural or psychological factors – place a person with SCD at potentially increasing risk of psychological disturbance, to the extent that consistently higher levels of diagnostic 'cases' are found among adults with SCD than healthy controls or those with other chronic illnesses. It may be that illness generally has greater potential for causing distress and anxiety in adults than in children because more personal responsibility is required for coping, which in adverse social and economic circumstances could precipitate mental or emotional disturbance by placing the individual under stress.

Sickle Cell Disease and the Adult Social World

So far we have been considering the 'environment' of the person with SCD in rather abstract terms. We end this chapter by looking in a more concrete way at two important areas in the lives of adults with SCD: (1) their social and family lives; and (2) their life at work. Aspects of both may be relevant to stress and adjustment in people with SCD, or may be restricted or complicated by the condition.

Friends and Family

In Black and Laws' (1986) study of adults with SCD in London, 86 per cent reported that SCD had affected their lives by restricting social activities, and 38 per cent reported that this restriction had a great impact on their lives. The wide range of activities that have been shown to precipitate sickling mean that many of the social and leisure activities so often taken for granted must be treated with caution by people with SCD. These include drinking alcohol, physical exertion, getting wet or chilled, swimming, high altitude, and even heavy meals. Young people, in whom peer group identification and exploratory, risk-taking behaviour may be significant aspects of personal development, might be expected to suffer more than older adults from exclusion from otherwise attractive activities. They might also be more likely to suffer socially as a result of embarrassment or inhibition about SCD, although stigmatization, or the fear of it, is felt widely among people with SCD. In Broome and Monroe's (1979) 'patient-perceived needs assessment' of 100 people with sickle cell disease in the Bay area of San Francisco, only 45 per cent of those questioned reported feeling 'good' or 'okay' when SCD was brought up with friends, and 20 per cent felt embarrassed or ashamed about having the condition.

Starting a Family

Possibly the most important choices to be made by adults with SCD relate to reproduction. Difficult decisions would arise earliest for those who intend to minimize the risk to their children by taking account of the genetic status of potential partners. Others may confront issues arising from the inheritance of SCD only after they have found a partner or started a pregnancy. Some women with SCD are very uncertain about their position in relation to having children of their own. Many may have been misinformed about the level of risk to themselves and their children. There are no studies of reproductive behaviour in relation to SCD, but in Modell, Ward, and Fairweather's (1980) study of families affected by thalassaemia trait, many couples discovered their risk only by producing a sick child, and knowledge of the risk of passing on thalassaemia caused them virtually to stop reproducing. In Black and Laws' (1986) interview study of people with SCD, all ten of those over the age of 25 were parents, and several had more than one child, but many of the women in their sample reported reluctance among male partners to have a blood test to ascertain whether they carried the trait.

The child of parents who both have SCD would be certain also to be affected, but this pairing would be unlikely to happen without the knowledge of the individuals concerned. Previously undetected presence in either parent of the trait for sickle cell would be much more likely to take parents by surprise, and where one person has either SCD or the sickle cell trait, the difference between partnering someone who does or does not have the trait is highly significant from a genetic point of view. The odds of illness for each child would be raised from 0 to 50 per cent where the first parent had SCD, and from 0 to 25 per cent where they had sickle cell trait.

All other things being equal, therefore, there is a considerable advantage for a person with SCD who intends to have children in finding a partner who does not have the trait. Of course, all other things are very rarely equal, so that the potential exists for very difficult choices. Some people may have had generally encouraging experiences of SCD and the prospect of a child with the illness may not frighten them. Others may feel strongly that the opportunity to prevent their children being exposed to SCD is worth taking the genetic status of a future partner into account. Couples, or potential couples, may find that they hold conflicting views on the question, or people without SCD may be reluctant to be tested for the trait through ignorance about SCD or for other reasons. Clearly, the genetic status of both partners needs to be known before fully informed decisions can be made about starting a family, although people vary in the extent to which they are prepared to make their choice of partner on such practical grounds.

Genetic Counselling

The main aim of genetic counselling is to allow people to make informed decisions about their health-related behaviour based on all the available information and options (Emery and Pullen, 1984). An important aspect of counselling relates to heredity, or risk in reproduction, but this is not the only thing to consider. Satcher (1976) has described the importance of dealing with self-concept and social relationships in counselling for SCD, which should also address personal physical and emotional health, and any aspects of life that are potentially affected by SCD. It is also worth emphasizing that the purpose of genetic counselling is not eugenic, that is, the elimination of 'undesirable' characteristics from the gene pool. Decisions made by people affected by SCD about whether or not to have children, whether to adopt, or whether to terminate a pregnancy in which SCD is indicated, might be expected in the long run to put selective pressure on the sickle cell gene, but any reduction in the incidence of SCD should be regarded as a side-effect of the primary purpose, which is to put individuals in the best position to make informed choices themselves about their health, and to ensure that individuals who are potentially affected by SCD begin to receive the best support available as early as possible.

Parenting

Mothers with SCD may require additional support because their own condition means that they may have to spend time at hospital, or because they are periodically unable to cope with looking after their children at home. Both formal and informal assistance with childcare would be expected to make a difference to the lives of women with SCD who have children, and childcare is among the most requested, and valued, form of support service among parents with SCD.

SCD clearly has the potential to affect parent–child relations. Where the parent but not the child has SCD it may be important for children to understand the nature of their parent's illness, and to have their own fears and uncertainties about the condition properly addressed. Where both parent and child are affected, it is important that children are not unduly influenced by their parents' experiences of the condition, which may be very different from their own. In almost every case, the potential impact of SCD is likely to be reduced by more accurate information and better understanding about SCD by all concerned, whether they are affected directly or share a family with someone who is.

Employment

By contrast with the situation in relation to medicine and health care, where people with SCD may be exposed to unnecessary suffering because the condition is not sufficiently well recognized or attended to, in the workplace they are more likely to be affected because the implications of SCD are exaggerated or are too widely generalized. People who have sickle cell trait may suffer particularly from erroneous views and beliefs about SCD. Konotey-Ahulu (1991), for example, has described how misleading scientific publications led to recommendations that people with the trait should not be employed as airline staff. In fact, people with sickle cell trait are always symptom-free when travelling in pressurized aircraft.

For those who have SCD, the level of employment-related problems depends upon the severity of symptoms and the extent to which they can be managed, the nature of the work in question, and the attitudes of the employer. Choice, or the scope for choice, of employment is a critical factor, for although the ability to maintain regular attendance at work may be an important consideration in employing a person with SCD (Franklin and Atkin, 1986), there is no reason why, in a suitable occupation, individuals with SCD should not be expected to perform as well as anyone. Such people are in almost every respect normal employees and can work to their full capacity during long periods of good health. The literature on SCD sometimes portrays individuals with SCD as suffering continuously with pain crises and a multitude of complications, but it is important to recognize that many are affected to a much lesser extent by clinical aspects of SCD, yet still experience discrimination in the workplace because of the condition. Dr Jeanne Smith (1973), for example, commented that:

> Those who are ill as a result of having sickle cell disease vary considerably in the severity of illness. There are physicians, teachers, nurses, and many other gainfully employed individuals who have the disease. These individuals are fortunate not because they have sickle cell disease but because they have managed to bypass the multiple impediments that society has put in the way of those with a chronic illness.

Employers need to understand the nature of SCD so that absence from work can be minimized. It is very important that potential restrictions of access to employment and of performance and satisfaction at work be kept to a minimum, for work is an important component of healthy adult adjustment. As Whitten and Fischoff (1974) have pointed out:

> The disease also imposes a sense of insecurity, for adults are quite aware that sickle cell anaemia may result in disqualification for a job or a dismissal after hiring. Because of the role of work and

self-sufficiency in the development of the individual's social identity, any factor that works against the acquisition and retention of a meaningful job has the potential for undermining or destroying a previously good psychosocial adjustment.

Suitable and Unsuitable Employment

People with SCD should avoid heavy manual work, exposure to extremes of temperature, exposure to lowered oxygen concentration, and work that cannot be interrupted to take fluids. Individuals may in addition be able to identify activities and situations that cause them problems and that they should avoid in seeking employment, and they should be aware of their own limitations. Vocational and career advisers have a role to play and should be aware of employment issues in relation to SCD.

For the vast majority of people with SCD, any restrictions to the type of work they can undertake would leave a wide range of acceptable occupations, including administration, artistic and light industrial work, and most of the professions. Many people with SCD perform highly skilled work, and many are attracted to medicine (Phillips, 1976). Many others, however, experience great difficulty in finding and keeping suitable jobs, and find that SCD places them at a significant disadvantage in the workplace. In Black and Laws' (1986) survey of people with SCD in Newham, London, nearly half (12 out of 26) of those over the age of 16 years were unemployed. Those who did work were in a variety of occupations, including two nurses and a dentist. Many of those interviewed reported terrible difficulties in getting and keeping work, and felt they were restricted in the type of work they could consider.

At Work

Once at work, the main problem facing people with SCD is the need for occasional absence. This would appear to be the most important factor in many people's apparent difficulty in achieving a stable employment record. Franklin and Atkin (1986) investigated the work history of 13 people with SCD in the West Midlands. They found that only three of the 11 people who had been employed had never lost their jobs because of problems related to SCD, and only one had been in employment for more than 3 years.

The main reason for losing jobs was repeated brief absences from work due to pain crises.

People with SCD may need to consider carefully whether or not to tell employers about their condition. Potential benefits would be sympathetic treatment and the opportunity to make arrangements to accommodate episodes of illness, but at the risk that employers would take a less sympathetic view and their job would be jeopardized. Those risks would be expected to be greater in lower paid, less skilled occupations where there are fewer protections for the employee.

There is in fact little systematic evidence about levels of knowledge and awareness of SCD among employers, managers, and in the workplace generally. Franklin and Atkin (1986) also interviewed 11 employers about their attitudes towards SCD. Over half (54 per cent) claimed to assess each employee individually on the basis of previous attendance records, medical history, and advice from the Occupational Health Service, and three reported that they had never had any problems with SCD and gave it no consideration in staff evaluation or selection. This rather rosy picture conflicted sharply with the perspective of their employees, many of whom had experienced problems at work in the past. From such a small sample it is impossible to make generalizations about the way that people with SCD are affected by company policies for recruitment and assessment, and studies would be welcome on the nature and prevalence of employment practices that present difficulties to people with SCD, and on associated individual attitudes and knowledge about SCD among managers and employers.

One option for a person with SCD and very serious problems at work in the UK is to register disabled. This would qualify them for employment under 'quota schemes' or in sheltered workshops, or for help with expenses, but the advantages to registration would depend on individual circumstances, and may not outweigh the disadvantages. A classification of 'disabled' could disqualify as well as qualify a person for some types of work, and might have social and psychological effects for someone who was healthy and able for much of the time.

Problems with work generally translate into problems with money. Many people with SCD live on low incomes or social security, yet may have to meet additional outgoings because of the very factors that limit their income. Financial constraints penalize the chronically ill more than the healthy, and people with SCD may suffer to a greater extent when, for financial reasons, they are not able to run a car, keep their central heating on for long periods of the year, or go on holiday, or when they have to live in damp or draughty accommodation, climb flights of stairs, or contend with disputes about registration as a citizen and perhaps face deportation.

Financial pressure is a key contributor to more general levels of stress and day-to-day coping hassles, and can often precipitate emotional and psychological problems. Conversely, a stimulating and satisfying working life can be a bulwark against assaults on self-confidence and self-image caused by disruption in other areas of life. Where SCD leads to underachievement and dissatisfaction in the workplace it has the potential to undermine positive adjustment more generally, although the extent to which employment is affected by SCD might in turn reflect the extent to which individuals have made successful adaptations to their condition. Either way, gainful employment is a central feature of healthy adult functioning and adjustment, and problems at work are frequently associated with indicators of distress in other areas of life. When things begin to go wrong at work for a person with SCD this might signal the onset of a vicious cycle of poverty, downward social mobility, distress, and maladjustment, whereas sensible and sensitive interventions in the workplace, by or on behalf of the individual concerned, might make the difference between an independent, coping style of adjustment and one characterized by dependence, low self-image, and feelings of helplessness.

7

Systems of Support in Sickle Cell Disease

Many of the findings described so far in this book indicate measures of a psychological or psychosocial nature that might benefit individuals and families affected by SCD. Some could be taken up by people on their own behalf. For example, relaxation techniques for the management of pain and self-monitoring of painful crises require only that the person is sufficiently motivated, well informed, and able to operate an individual programme. Organized interventions such as support groups could also be set up by families or individuals acting on their own behalf. Most measures, however, would require a more co-ordinated initiative on the part of those who are involved professionally in the provision of health, education, and social services. These all have a role to play in care for SCD. Some services are already well established, and others are in earlier stages of development. In almost every case, their effectiveness could be improved by increasing the level of uptake, by tailoring services to meet particular needs, and by integrating the provision of different services. In many cases, there is a need for the development and evaluation of new or innovatory services.

The first purpose of this chapter is to review existing service provision for SCD in the UK, and to explain the roles played by different health care and social service professionals. We shall also consider how these services are likely to develop in the future, and how such changes could most usefully accommodate the findings that have emerged from psychosocial research on SCD.

Medical Services

Medical services are the front line of support for patients with SCD, for without adequate medical provision other forms of support and assistance are unlikely to be effective. However, maximizing the benefits obtained from medical services can also depend upon other forms of support that are at present underdeveloped and underco-ordinated by comparison with medical services.

Hospitals are the main focus for the delivery of medical services, with community-based services playing a subsidiary role at present. Few patients with SCD avoid hospitalization altogether for complications of their condition, and a diagnosis of SCD is usually made in hospital. There are 23 Sickle Cell and Thalassaemia Centres in the UK, many of which are also based in hospitals (*see* Appendix 1), and these centres are the primary medium for the integration and co-ordination of services for supportive assistance in SCD. In the USA, there are 10 Comprehensive Sickle Cell Centres (*see* Appendix 2) and a new directory of support groups has just been produced (Nash *et al.*, 1993).

Medical services for people affected by SCD can be divided into three broad categories. The first relates to the identification of individuals at risk through screening, followed by counselling. The second category concerns specific medical interventions that might constitute potential cures for SCD. Generally speaking, the procedures involved are limited, at an early stage of development, and offer uncertain outcomes. The third, and by far the largest and most important, covers mainstream medical support, whose aim is to prevent, delay and minimize the complications caused by SCD.

Screening, Testing, and Counselling

Sickle cell disease can be diagnosed at or before birth by routine screening methods. Haemoglobin electrophoresis is used to identify haemoglobin phenotypes (HbAA, AS, SC, SS, etc.) in the blood from birth. Prenatal diagnosis on the fetus can be carried out by DNA studies using chorionic villus sampling (CVS) or amniotic fluid cells from amniocentesis. CVS is now generally performed at between 10 and 16 weeks through the abdominal wall. A later diagnosis (*circa* 20–22 weeks) can also be made by testing fetal blood taken by chordocentesis. All these prenatal tests carry a risk of causing a miscarriage.

In spite of our ability to detect SCD safely and reliably from birth, the diagnosis is in many cases made only when a child is first brought to hospital in crisis. The implication of this is that children are exposed to avoidable suffering and risk of early death because the implementation of preventive measures was delayed. Bainbridge *et al.* (1985) reported that over 30 per cent of deaths occurred before a diagnosis was made. Powars (1989) has shown that facilitating prompt parental education and early treatment for the child with prophylactic penicillin can improve the survival rate of children with SCD. As we shall see, there is a very strong case for improving neonatal screening programmes in order to identify every individual who could be affected by SCD as early in their life as possible.

At present, screening services are variable, with different policies followed in different areas (Prashar, Anionwu, and Brozovic, 1985). For example, Potrykus (1991) interviewed SCD workers from six London districts. Despite the fact that all six districts contain large Afro-Caribbean communities, provision of screening services was patchy and poor. Only three districts screened all babies at birth for SCD, although most screened all pregnant women. Selective screening, targeted at people of African or Afro-Caribbean origin, is the most widely followed screening policy in Britain. Decisions about what screening policy to adopt are made by applying a cost–benefit analysis based on the size of the at-risk population and the extent to which it is diluted genetically by those of North European origin.

A cost–benefit analysis of this kind would involve weighing the chances of failing to detect cases of SCD and the legal costs of this failure against the extra resources that would be required to prevent this happening. In fact, such analyses may be short-sighted even in economic terms, because, in addition to improving the chances of survival and quality of life of sufferers, early diagnosis can help to avoid potentially costly demands on medical resources at a later stage. Demands on emergency services and admissions to hospital, for example, could be reduced by early implementation of preventive care and support.

The main problem with a selective screening programme is the difficulty in selecting who to screen, because it is important to screen everyone who is not of pure North European origin. Selection for screening cannot be based simply on the language, nationality, or appearance of individuals, but requires close questioning by sensitive and knowledgeable staff, although in fact it is often undertaken by relatively junior, inexperienced workers. Selective screening is least effective in multicultural societies, where mixed marriages increase the likelihood of at-risk individuals not being screened because they are 'white' in appearance.

Testing for SCD should always be accompanied by counselling, one of the most important aspects of which is parental education following neonatal diagnosis. Majorie Ferguson, a nurse counsellor with the George Marsh Sickle Cell Centre in Haringey, North London, has described the role of the counsellor in supporting and advising parents whose child has been positively diagnosed for sickle cell disease (Ferguson, 1991). She aims to see the family at least three times during the first 3 months of the new baby's life; a period when it will usually be symptom-free.

The process begins by breaking the news of the test result to the parents as soon as it is available, and providing information about the nature of the condition. This is followed by a home visit some weeks later, after the parents' initial reaction to the news. A home visit gives the counsellor an opportunity to assess the coping skills, attitudes, and interpersonal dynamics of the family, and to instruct the parents in practical ways to care for the child in order to prevent and minimize harm.

The next contact with the family would be at the Sickle Cell Centre, where parents have the opportunity to meet others in the same position, perhaps watch a video about SCD, and communicate their experiences so far. The Sickle Cell Centre should be a gateway into various medical and support services, including the family doctor, the paediatric clinic, family support groups, and any other local services, and can provide a focus for the kind of integrated package of preventive care, support, and response to crisis that has been advocated by many workers in the area.

Specific Medical Interventions

Luzzatto and Goodfellow (1989) have described five basic treatment strategies for sickle cell disease. These are: (1) antisickling agents; (2) vasoactive drugs; (3) promotion of the persistence of fetal haemoglobin; (4) bone marrow transplantation; and (5) gene therapies. The first three approaches have more or less failed so far to provide a reliable and effective way to prevent sickling crises. Many antisickling drugs are under investigation (Davis, Vichinsky, and Lubin, 1980), and although some extracts have been reported to reverse sickling *in vitro* and to reduce SCD pain (Adekile *et al.*, 1990), they are at present experimental and do not constitute a cure. Hydroxyurea appears to increase fetal haemoglobin production and decrease the rate of haemolysis, and has been reported to reduce the frequency and severity of painful episodes (Rodgers, Dover and Noguchi, 1990). Clinical trials are in progress to determine its optimal dosage and long-term safety, but the drug is associated with impaired fertility, teratogenic risk, and may have long-term carcinogenic side-effects.

Bone Marrow Transplant

Bone marrow transplantation (BMT) can cure SCD and thalas-saemia. The procedure involves replacing abnormal haematopoie-tic stem cells (the cells that produce SS red blood cells, white cells, and platelets) with normal cells from a matched donor who has a non-symptomatic haemoglobin genotype. A successful operation will allow the patient to produce normal haemoglobin for the rest of their life, but there are significant risks, including rejection, infection, and 'graft versus host disease', all of which are poten-tially fatal.

For β Thalassaemia Major, Lucarelli *et al.* (1990) have reported that in good-risk patients below 16 years, 94 per cent survive free of symptoms for at least 3 years after transplantation. The first successful BMT for β Thalassaemia Major was recorded in 1982 (Thomas *et al.*, 1982), and the operation is now becoming increas-ingly common, especially in Italy, where more than 500 trans-plants have taken place.

A decision to procede with BMT involves weighing the risks of early mortality from an unsuccessful transplant and long-term side-effects against the increase in quality of life, which is the prize of success. The decision is much more difficult to make with SS than with β Thalassaemia Major, because the severity of sickle cell anaemia is much more variable (Kodish *et al.*, 1990). Factors affecting the likelihood of successful transplantation and the 'man-ageability' of the condition without transplantation all need to be considered in deciding whether the operation would be in the best interests of the patient. The first BMT for SCD was performed on an 8-year-old girl who also had acute leukaemia (Johnson *et al.*, 1984). Since then, more than 50 patients with SCD have received transplants, and Vermylen *et al.* (1988), and Kirkpatrick, Barrios, and Humbert (1991) have reviewed the results of the first 21 cases, which were broadly encouraging. Most of the recipients were still alive some 3 to 5 years later.

The critical issue for the doctor practising BMT is the selection of patients (Davies, 1993). Availability of a suitable matched donor is an obviously important factor. Best results are achieved when the patient and donor's tissue (HLA) are identical, which is most likely in siblings or, ideally, identical twins. The patient's own prognosis must also be taken into account. Normally, one would select the most severe cases for a new and risky procedure. However, clinical history is not always a reliable guide to pros-pects in the future for patients with SCD. BMT is most successful in young patients who have a serious prognosis but not such a serious clinical history that they have already suffered significant organ damage. The difficulty arises in estimating at an early stage the likely future severity of the condition. This is not necessarily related to the severity of complications that have been experienced during the first years of life. Assessment and prediction of severity is therefore more than an academic research issue (*see* Chapter 2), for accurate and predictive indices of severity would be invaluable clinically. Nagel (1991) has argued that a 10 per cent mortality risk for transplantation (the current ball-park estimate) would be acceptable in cases where there have been complications involving the central nervous system (strokes) or where there have been repeated episodes of acute chest syndrome, both of which are associated with poor prognosis.

The decision about whether or not to attempt a BMT is therefore a difficult and sensitive one. Various factors must be weighed in the balance, including the chances of success of the operation, the patient's prognosis, and how the patient perceives their quality of life without the operation. Cost may be another consideration. The operation is expensive (estimated at around $115 000 by Welch and Larson (1989) or $10 000 per additional year of life, on average), but Kirkpatrick *et al.* (1991) argue that it works out cheaper than long-term blood transfusions and iron chelation therapy. In addition, the possibility of the development of a safer treatment or 'cure' in the future cannot be ruled out, although at present this seems unlikely. Many of these factors are clearly difficult to quantify, and 'quality of life' is an area in which medical experts may not be best placed to make assessments on behalf of the individual concerned.

From an ethical point of view, there would be few misgivings about presenting an informed choice between risking the procedure and continuing to manage the condition, if the choice could be made by the patient with appropriate counselling. In fact, this is almost never the case because transplantation offers the best chances of success when performed early in life, so that the decision would fall instead to the parent or guardian of a young patient. Variations in the quality of health care available also mean that some families have a more difficult and painful choice to make than others. In some circumstances, parents might opt to risk transplantation because they feel that adequate provision for a child with SCD cannot be guaranteed for social or economic reasons. The pioneering work on BMT in SCD involved five children from Zaire who were taken to Belgium for transplants because the doctors concerned judged that proper medical care could not be secured for them in their own country (Vermylen *et al.*, 1988). As in many other areas of medicine, future sufferers benefit from the risks taken by those in disadvantaged groups.

Gene therapy

Gene therapy means reversing the alteration in the genetic codes that are the cause of SCD. The procedure would involve transferring HbA β globin genes to the bone marrow cells of the affected individual *in vitro*. If the transfer was successful then the bone marrow cells would be retransfused into the patient after ablating the rest of the bone marrow cells. Luzzatto and Goodfellow (1989) have suggested that the ideal way of conducting gene therapy would involve replacing the mutated β globin gene by homologous recombination. However, there is much to be learnt about the biology of stem cells before gene therapy would constitute a realistic treatment option.

Mainstream Medical Services

In addition to those medical interventions that aim to reverse the primary characteristics of SCD, there is an important role for more routine medical support and intervention in order to minimize secondary effects of the condition, prevent complications arising where possible, and deal with crises and episodic complications as they occur. People with SCD are also, of course, as likely as anyone else to require medical services because they are involved in accidents, become pregnant and give birth, or require medical treatment for reasons unrelated to SCD. Sickle cell disease can affect the type of treatment they should receive, or may indicate that certain cautions should be observed when particular procedures are used.

The average patient with SCD, if there is such a thing, is likely to encounter various medical services during their life. The range of medical complications associated with the condition is steadily increasing because as people with SCD live longer they run into complications of the condition that previous sufferers did not survive to encounter. In SCD, as in health care generally, increased survival rates and life expectancy due to successful interventions in one area have led to increased demand for treatments in others. In a sense, many of the medical problems faced by people with

SCD are the result of the success of medicine in extending their life expectancy, for the 'natural history' of the condition is that 50 per cent would die before the age of 20. In the 1940s there was even speculation about whether SS was really related to the sickle cell trait, because although the trait was very common in Africa, the disease was very rarely encountered because of the very low survival rate of affected children.

Now, however, 95 per cent of children with SCD survive to 20 years of age, and around 60 per cent survive to middle age. Children who once died of infections are now saved by immunization and antibiotics, and early deaths caused by sequestration crises can be avoided. Strokes, loss of renal function, and cardiopulmonary complications are now the biggest killers, whilst painful crises and leg ulcers are important non-lethal complications. There is, however, scope for considerable improvement in the delivery of medical expertise to sufferers of SCD. In particular, various measures could be instituted earlier on a preventive basis, rather than as a response to crises. Piomelli (1991), for example, has called for a regime of 'active preventive intervention' in order to make the best use of existing medical capacity to combat the complications caused by SCD.

Accident and Emergency Departments

Prompt action and adequate analgesia are essential for the treatment of painful crises. Haemoglobinopathy cards with the address of the nearest clinic and the number of the patient's medical records, issued by Sickle Cell Centres, could help to facilitate this. However, many hospitals seem unable to respond optimally when people with SCD present in crisis to Accident and Emergency Departments. Patients have reported a lack of sympathy from some doctors and nurses, and long waiting times (sometimes up to 5 hours) before receiving treatment (Midence et al., 1992a). Wyatt (1988) has pointed out that although some medical doctors and nurses may remember some of their molecular biology, most of them regard SCD as a rare tropical condition and have seldom met a sufferer or know how to respond to their problems.

Some efforts are being made to improve emergency services. With the co-operation of a large multidisciplinary group, the Brent Sickle Cell Centre at the Central Middlesex Hospital in London has developed an 'Adult Painful Sickle Cell Crisis Protocol/Care Plan'.

This protocol includes the participation of receptionists, emergency unit nurses, junior doctors, ward nurses, consultant haematologists, and the nurse specialists from the Sickle Cell Centre. Pain management is protocol-driven, with clear quality guidelines; tests and procedures are carried out in a planned sequence; discharge planning starts early; and patients leave the hospital with clear, written information about the treatment that they received.

Medical Services in the Community

General practitioners (GPs) are in the community frontline and could potentially play a major role in health education, genetic counselling, prompt intervention in cases of infection, and as a gateway to specialized clinics. There is a good case for GPs to become more involved in the care of people with SCD in an advisory, supportive, and preventative role. However, several obstacles stand in the way of an increased role for GPs in the care and treatment of SCD. Many would require additional training and support in order to be able to respond effectively to problems associated with SCD and to identify those complications that indicate prompt referral to specialist care. The burden on GPs is presently increasing in Britain because of the general shift towards care in the community. Many GPs are also wary of patients complaining of pain (Bell, 1991). They are sometimes approached by drug users seeking analgesics, and their experiences of these people, typically described as manipulative and disruptive, have led to some unwillingness to prescribe for the relief of pain, so that patients with SCD may not receive the most sympathetic reception (Foster, 1991).

Because of these factors, GPs are probably giving a less than optimal service to their patients with SCD. In Black and Laws' (1986) survey, only four out of 44 people with SCD interviewed did not use the services of their GP, but over one-third of those who did reported that their GP was not understanding of their problems with SCD. The most common problems reported were a lack of knowledge among GPs about SCD and problems with obtaining prescriptions. Studies on GPs' knowledge of the haemoglobinopathies have also indicated a lack of awareness and low levels of involvement in the care of people with SCD (Shickle and May, 1989). Unfamiliarity with the literature on prescribed medication amongst GPs is a major limitation in the provision of a high quality service and the implementation of haemoglobinopathy prevention programmes (Cummins, Heuschkel, and Davies, 1991).

There is also a strong argument for extending screening programmes from hospitals to community-based services. Some infants are missed by hospital neonatal screening programmes because they were born at home or in a different hospital (Miller *et al.*, 1990), whereas community-based programmes allow results to be cross-checked with birth notifications.

Population screening for sickle cell trait is straightforward in technical terms but, as Modell (1991) has pointed out, clinical geneticists working in hospitals would not be best placed to take on the public health tasks of organizing large-scale genetic screening and counselling. Instead, 'community genetics' or 'community haematology' would be needed, in collaboration with experts in public health medicine. The general requirements of a programme of population screening for genetic carrier status of hereditary conditions have been summarized by the World Health Organization (1985). Most of these relate to the integration and co-ordination of technical and information systems. The Royal College of Physicians (1989) has already considered existing community genetic services, and identified problems in the delivery of such services. These also related mostly to the integration and co-ordination of separate systems and services. A community-based genetic screening programme of this kind would offer a realistic opportunity to minimize the incidence of SCD in a similar way to the approach which has been adopted for cystic fibrosis.

Screening programmes could be run at GPs' surgeries and health centres, well-women clinics, infertility clinics, and community centres locally and nationally; health visitors could also become involved. However, the impact and cost-effectiveness of screening programmes at diverse agencies and sites in the community would depend on the extent to which information could be shared and activities co-ordinated. This would probably require the setting up of a centralized agency through which information could be channelled, in order to avoid duplication of work and to ensure that test results were followed up promptly and effectively with the appropriate action. However, such a programme raises issues of confidentiality, which would need to be addressed if the system were to achieve the necessary levels of confidence and co-operation on the part of the public.

Staff Knowledge and Attitudes

Illnesses affect subsets of the population, and those involved in the care of affected people need to have some awareness of non-medical factors that may influence the experiences and responses of patients in relation to their condition and the treatment they receive. This is especially true when particular ethnic groups are affected by an illness, for matters of culture, tradition, and language all play a role in determining the extent to which patients are adversely affected by aspects of a medical condition and the different treatment regimes to which they may be subjected. The less a clinician is aware of these factors, the less well placed he or she is to make realistic clinical judgements about the patients' situation and to provide adequate and realistic care.

There is a growing body of evidence that black people in Britain receive a quantitatively and qualitatively worse service than white people (National Association of Health Authorities, 1988). At all levels, the response of the Health Service to ethnic issues has been characterized by a stereotyped view of black people and their needs, in which black *people*, rather than the conditions from which they suffer, are seen as a problem (Mohammed, 1991). Nash (1977) has suggested that effective treatment of SCD patients requires health care professionals to become aware of their own attitudes towards patients' race and culture. In relation to the families of children with SCD, Jackson (1972) commented that: 'A lack of understanding of the condition combined with frequent abuse or apathy by those from whom they sought help compounded the awesome burden of families with these chronically ill children'.

The effects on patients of inapropriate attitudes on the part of medical staff may be compounded in many cases by a lack of basic knowledge about SCD. Charache and Davies (1991) used a multiple-choice questionnaire to assess knowledge about the management of SCD amongst house officers in both the US and the UK; US house officers produced higher average scores than their UK counterparts. More than half of the respondents in both countries thought that sickle cell trait produced mild anaemia, and more than 10 per cent did not know the risks of having a child with sickle cell anaemia if both parents are carriers.

The aspect of treatment most likely to be influenced by attitudes and opinions held by medical professionals is relief from pain. Those who specialize in the treatment of SCD pain (Brookoff, 1992) have described how care often falls far short of the general medical principle that patients in pain have a legitimate right to analgesia, and how people with SCD are often received less than sympathetically when requesting medication for pain. Black and Laws (1986) documented many accounts by patients with SCD of unsympathetic treatment by doctors in casualty departments. The most common complaints involved delays before administering analgesia, which were caused by searches for medical notes, waiting 'to see whether the pain went away', performing investigations such as X-rays, or questioning the mother about possible child abuse. On the wards, staff had apparently often failed to recognize the severity of SCD pain or had questioned its authenticity, and in some cases parents reported having to instruct medical staff on what to do. Many of these problems could be reduced by improvements in the level of knowledge about SCD among medical staff, and the need for more inservice training in haemoglobinopathies for health visitors, nurses, medical doctors, and health care professionals in general have been highlighted by various authors (Shickle and May, 1989; France-Dawson, 1990; Cummins *et al.*, 1991; Anionwu, 1992).

People with SCD are probably not the only ones to suffer because of conservative prescribing practices for chronic pain. Dahl *et al.* (1988) have concluded that undertreatment of pain in hospitals is largely due to three factors: (1) inadequate knowledge among health professionals about pain and its treatment; (2) excessive fear of addiction on the part of health professionals and the public; and (3) underuse of existing pain management techniques. People with SCD are likely to suffer on all three counts because of the episodic and unpredictable nature of their pain, the low levels of knowledge and awareness of SCD among many medical doctors, and the often poor appreciation by professionals of cultural attitudes in the affected black community. On the question of addiction to pain-killing drugs, it is right that doctors should be aware of the risk of contributing to the drug problem but, as McQuay (1989) has pointed out, it is unjust to deprive patients of pain relief because of the fear that medical supplies may go astray or that drugs would be misused.

Lack of knowledge about SCD and the treatment of pain, and generally unsympathetic attitudes towards people with SCD, all have the potential to undermine effective care and support for the condition. As we look around for ways in which psychological interventions could improve the management of SCD, one area in which changes could be made is among the health professionals themselves. Nobody can know everything, but there is a need for

114

greater awareness of SCD generally among hospital doctors and for an improved knowledge of pain management among those who work with SCD. Low levels of awareness among doctors of the cultures, religious beliefs, and social attitudes in the communities affected by SCD are also common. Institutionalized racism and inappropriate attitudes and behaviours on the part of medical and other staff continue to affect the care provided for people with SCD, and these issues need to be addressed before the management of SCD could reach the standards which are possible.

Non-Medical Services

Non-medical services are important for two reasons. First, the patient benefits from support and services that complement their medical treatment by providing a more detailed assessment of needs, explaining the choices of treatment available and their implications, and attending to concerns and anxieties raised by patients about their condition and about their medical treatment. As Gaston (1973) pointed out: 'Through effective co-ordination and communication by a multi-faceted team, improvement of the quality of life with a realistic outlook for the future can be achieved.'

Second, the provision of integrated, multidisciplinary services in support of primary medical treatment promotes good husbandry of medical resources by facilitating better compliance with treatment regimes, monitoring the outcomes of treatment, and helping to ensure that, where medical interventions are necessary, they are applied in good time. Vichinsky *et al.* (1982) evaluated a multidisciplinary psychosocial programme in the US which included support groups, self-hypnosis, psychosocial assessment and follow-up, psychotherapy, a 24-hour hot-line, and home visits by nurses, with elements of the package tailored to the needs of individuals. The programme had a marked effect on demand for centralized hospital services, reducing hospital admissions by 48 per cent, and emergency visits by 58 per cent by comparison with levels observed before the programme was introduced.

Vavasseur (1977) has described some of the methods used at the Comprehensive Sickle Cell Centre in Los Angeles. There the medical social worker plays a key role in counselling and support, taking referrals from inpatient wards, nurses, and staff throughout the medical centre, and counselling patients at home, in the clinic, in the centre, or on the wards. Among the benefits of this service is that patients find it less necessary to have a 'medical' complaint in order to get supportive attention, so that the number of visits to emergency rooms by patients with vague complaints for which there is no clinical basis can be minimized.

Sickle Cell Centres

Establishing sickle cell centres is probably the most effective and cost-effective way of delivering comprehensive care and support to people with SCD and the at-risk community. They are a relatively recent development in Europe, but now play a central role in integrating the services available to SCD sufferers in many countries. The first centres were established in the US in the early 1970s, whilst in the UK the Brent Sickle Cell and Thalassaemia Centre was set up in 1979, to be followed by several others, including City and Hackney, Islington, Lambeth, Haringey, Liverpool, and Manchester, in the 1980s.

Prashar *et al.* (1985) have described seven main functions of a sickle cell centre. These are: (1) to initiate, organize and co-ordinate screening and counselling facilities; (2) to conduct antenatal screening and counselling and prenatal diagnosis; (3) to conduct neonatal screening, parental education, and organize follow-up programmes; (4) to provide a social, education, and employment advisory and support service; (5) to provide an information service for healthcare professionals, patients, and their families, and the community in general; (6) to run inservice training of nurse-counsellors; and (7) to keep a register of patients with SCD. However, many sickle cell centres in this country are struggling to meet these goals. The training of haemoglobinopathy nurse-counsellors has been ignored by some Health Authorities, and counselling courses have been organized by only a few centres. Most centres now have some mainstream NHS funding but financial uncertainty affects their capacity to provide and develop the full range of services required by their clients (Prashar *et al.*, 1985). There is also a need for more centres in the UK, especially in those areas where the incidence of SCD is highest.

Educational Support

In Chapter 4 we looked at how the education of children with SCD can be affected in various ways by their condition, the most

116

important of which was absence from school because of pain crises and hospital attendances. There is therefore a strong case for including teachers and schools in the 'package' of integrated services made available to those affected by SCD. Attendance and performance at school are among the most important ways in which the lives of children with SCD can be disrupted, and flexible arrangements to compensate for the effects of enforced absence from school, coupled with increased knowledge and more appropriate attitudes among teachers, could help to alleviate the educational limitations that are often imposed by the condition. Shapiro (1989) has called for greater understanding of the effects of pain crises on school attendance and academic achievement in order to formulate appropriate educational policies, but some basic measures have already been shown to be effective. Walco and Dampier (1987), for example, found that education among children with SCD could be promoted by increased liaison between patients, their families, and their teachers. Crawford (1991) has highlighted the role of the school nurse, who could play a vital role by liaising with educational authorities and families to monitor the progress of children with SCD.

There is also a vital role for education to play by increasing awareness and knowledge of the condition among sufferers and non-sufferers. Jackson (1973) has suggested that:

> By far the most important facet of any service program in sickle cell is that of creating an awareness of the disorder, followed by presentation of accurate information. Emphasis has been placed on providing a comprehensive program with education as the foundation.

Screening programmes in schools could serve a dual function of identifying those who are potentially affected by SCD and illustrating more general genetic principles. In fact, screening for thalassaemia is already offered in high school in some parts of Italy (Bianco et al., 1984).

Social Services

Social workers have a vitally important role to play in the care and support of those affected by SCD because adequate provision for financial, housing, and other basic needs are prerequisite conditions for the optimal management of a chronic illness, and because black people are at greater risk generally of finding them-

117

selves in adverse social and economic circumstances (Oppenheim, 1990). Brown (1984), for example, found that black people in Britain lived in smaller properties, on average, than white people, and were more likely to experience overcrowding. Areas in which people with SCD would benefit from social worker support include help with heating, damp and insulation; holidays (McCalman (1990) described how only eight out of 34 black people caring for a disabled relative had been on holiday since they began caring); home help and childcare; the costs of medicines (unlike those with epilepsy, diabetes, and other conditions, people with SCD are not exempt from prescription charges); and obtaining benefits, such as disability allowance, for which they may qualify. A high proportion of children with SCD are in single parent families with various social and economic needs and, where these are not met, the individual and the family are placed at a disadvantage in their attempts to cope with illness.

In the Community

The community is a potentially valuable source of informal care and support from which people with chronic illnesses may benefit to varying extents. Help may come from the extended family, the neighbourhood, cultural and religious groups, and a wide range of other contacts and networks with whom affected persons may be in touch. One of the most significant areas of contact in the community is with other sufferers.

People with SCD and their families are themselves part of the community, and their own resources and skills could be much better harnessed (Anionwu, 1977). There is little doubt, for example, that support groups of patients and parents are effective in improving the quality of their own lives and reducing the demands they make on statutory services. Bringing people and families affected by SCD into contact with one another can be regarded as the most minimal, low-cost intervention possible, and Ferguson (1991) has pointed out how parents of children with SCD benefit from meeting other parents in a similar position with greater experience.

Support groups for people with chronic illness and their families have included multifamily discussion groups (Gonzalez, Steinglass, and Reiss, 1989), task-oriented groups (Conyard *et al.*, 1980), and ego-supportive groups (Markovitz, 1984). The main aims of such groups are educational and supportive, and their activities

118

usually focus on sharing information and allowing the expression and exploration of feelings. LePontois (1975) reported on a long-term support group for adolescent females with SCD. The group helped to prevent isolation, alienation, and dependency during the period when the young women were separating from their families.

The existence of an extensive network of informal support among the community of people affected by SCD should not be taken for granted. Atkin and Rollings (1992) have pointed out that the notion of the extended black family is not borne out by the evidence from surveys of African and Caribbean families in Britain, which show that many black people in this country live alone or have only infrequent contact with their families. Older black people may be at particular risk of social isolation (Fenton, 1987).

For the Future

Two broad themes emerge from this reading of existing service provision for SCD. The first is the need to bring larger numbers of those who are, or who could be, affected by SCD into contact with organized, professional services. The second is the need to integrate services more closely in order to deliver a more comprehensive, flexible, and responsive package of care to those who could benefit.

Prashar *et al.* (1985) have identified three areas for service improvements. The first is for services delivered directly to those affected, including more screening of the at-risk population and registration of people with SCD to allow for follow-up services and research. The second is in the field of professional awareness, which could be improved through in-service training and haemoglobinopathy courses. The third is education of the public, which is needed to reduce stigmatization and prejudice to which people with SCD may be exposed in various areas of life, and which stem largely from ignorance and misconceptions about the nature of SCD. In relation to the first of these, it has been suggested (Davies, 1988a) that community screening should be available on a self-referral basis as well as on medical request, and that there should be routine antenatal programmes in all urban districts.

British screening services have been developing over the past decade but are still highly variable nationally. Although the role

119

of sickle cell centres and haemoglobinopathy nurse-counsellors is being recognized (Anionwu, 1989b), a major problem for the development of counselling services is that there is no career structure for nurse-counsellors, whose present salary structure does not recognize their specialist expertise (Davies, 1988a). However, Prashar *et al.* (1985, p. 50) concluded that the most significant obstacles to the provision of better SCD services were that: '... there are no central guidelines and that no resources have been made available either centrally or locally'.

Clearly, political will and adequate funding are prerequisites for improvements in service provision, for one of the most important needs in this area is simply for *more* services generally. More haemoglobinopathy counselling courses, more sickle cell centres, and more nurse-counsellors are all needed to develop comprehensive haemoglobinopathy services and deliver a more even distribution of health care to those at risk.

8

Overview and Conclusions

The purpose of this book has been to provide an overview of SCD from a psychosocial perspective, together with a comprehensive review of the relevant empirical evidence. In this final chapter we first summarize the current state of knowledge in this area. We go on to consider worthwhile directions for future research of this kind. Lastly, we step back from the psychological or psychosocial perspective to consider some of the issues raised by SCD in a wider cultural and political context.

Findings to Date

The picture of SCD presented in the psychological literature has changed over time, as it has for most chronic illnesses. Early studies, informed partly by the need to increase awareness of SCD, tended to emphasize the potential seriousness of the condition and focused on maladjustment and other difficulties experienced by some affected people. Accumulated evidence about the resilience of many individuals and families, coupled with more sophisticated methods of sampling and measurement, has meant that more recent work has generally presented a rather less gloomy picture of the psychosocial implications of SCD. Emphasis has also shifted from potential maladjustment to positive aspects of coping and ways in which the provision and delivery of supportive care could be improved, so that the scope for findings to feed back into benefits to affected people has also increased.

Risk of Maladjustment and Psychopathology

The balance of evidence suggests that the overall risk of serious psychological dysfunction attributable solely to SCD is marginal. Studies of children have produced mixed results over a range of

121

measures, but appear to show that adolescent boys experience the highest levels of behavioural and psychological problems. Studies of adults appear to indicate a link between SCD and symptoms of depression and other psychological problems, but it is not clear to what extent the types of problem observed constitute genuine psychopathologies, or to what extent SCD is responsible for their appearance. In line with findings on chronic illness more generally, the majority of those affected by SCD show few signs of psychological disturbance, and many cope remarkably well. The most important theme to emerge from this area of investigation is variability in outcome, with numerous factors, both known and unknown, contributing to poorer adjustment among a significant minority of those potentially at risk. Illness severity is a poor predictor of adjustment generally, which seems to be influenced to a greater extent by socio-economic and lifestyle factors. More favourable social and economic circumstances, easier access to higher quality supportive services, and more positive individual styles of coping have all been shown to be associated with better outcomes in terms of psychological problems and adjustment to the limitations imposed by SCD.

The ways in which variables like these interact to influence coping and adjustment is by no means clear, but stress is probably an important mediating factor. Wallander and colleagues (Varni and Wallander, 1988) have suggested that families of chronically ill children are at greater risk of maladjustment because they are exposed to a greater number of stressful situations. Similarly, Burlew, Evans, and Oler (1989) have pointed out that the more psychosocial stressors within the family, the less effectively the affected individual and their family will be able to cope with the condition.

Positive Adaptation

In view of the evidence that many people with SCD cope remarkably well, much of the more recent work on SCD has been concerned with identifying and understanding positive coping mechanisms. Several studies have shown that positive styles of thinking about and responding to SCD were associated with lower levels of distress, inactivity and medical requirements during pain crises (Gil et al., 1991; Thompson et al., 1992). Such findings go some way towards explaining the variability in outcomes among individuals in similar circumstances, and factors of this kind are

122

probably important influences on levels of perceived stress, but in spite of a great deal of qualitative research in this area it is still not possible to offer a clear practical guide to potentially useful behavioural strategies. Self-monitoring and diary-keeping have been reported to be useful for some people, but have not been subject to systematic investigation. The role of family interactions and relationships also appear to be important factors in successful adaptation to SCD, with more supportive and expressive styles of family interaction associated with better coping and adaptation among affected individuals. Knowledge about these aspects of family functioning could therefore provide clues to the way that family dynamics contribute to positive adaptation.

From the point of view of promoting coping strategies, the most useful starting point would probably be behavioural methods for the control of pain, although any technique that assisted in the transfer of control over the condition from medicine and institutions to the individual would be expected to promote more positive adaptation and perceived freedom from the impositions of SCD. At a practical level, it is much less clear what types of strategy would be most effective for which individuals, and how potentially effective coping strategies could be taught and maintained.

Pain

The experience and management of pain belong at the heart of any behavioural or psychological analysis of SCD. Pain has been shown to be the most distressing feature of the condition from the point of view of affected people, and accounts for a good deal of the disruption to lifestyle and limitations imposed by SCD.

The characteristics of SCD pain (variable in intensity and frequency, episodic, and unpredictable) could almost have been designed to maximize its psychological impact, and the experience of pain probably contributes significantly to depression, anxiety, and other psychological problems sometimes associated with SCD. It seems highly likely that a great deal of SCD pain is undertreated with appropriate analgesia, partly because it is so variable and unpredictable, but behavioural methods for pain control have also been neglected. Hypnosis and biofeedback have been shown to be effective in controlling pain in rather limited trials, but it is not clear to what extent such techniques, which usually require specialized equipment or instruction, could benefit

123

larger numbers of affected people. Given the nature of SCD pain, considerable scope should exist for behavioural programmes aiming to help individuals to avoid painful episodes and to respond promptly and appropriately at the onset of pain crises. Such programmes would need to be tailored to individual needs and abilities, and to be compatible with existing arrangements for pain management, the most important of which is analgesia.

There is some evidence that much SCD pain is medically under-treated at present because of professional reluctance to use opiates for chronic, intermittent, and non-malignant pain. There are good reasons for caution in the use of drugs of potential abuse, and it would be irresponsible to advocate more liberal prescribing of opiates without appropriate safeguards against creating dependency and contributing to the availability of opiates on the street market. However, much of the anxiety and distress associated with SCD pain can be attributed to uncertainty on the part of sufferers about the quality of pain relief they can expect to receive, and many of the reasons for inadequate analgesia probably relate to lack of knowledge and expertise about SCD, pain control, the pharmacology of analgesics, and the risk of dependency on analgesic medication among non-specialists. The effectiveness of both behavioural and pharmacological approaches to pain management would be maximized by integrating both elements in individual protocols; behavioural programmes would be expected to be followed more consistently where individuals were confident that adequate analgesia would be available where necessary, and medical staff would feel more comfortable about using drugs for the relief of SCD pain where this formed part of an overall treatment strategy including the monitoring and prevention of painful crises, and non-pharmacological control of pain where possible.

Service Provision

A good deal of current research on SCD is examining family relationships, coping skills and personal adjustment in relation to the quality and availability of medical and social services. It hardly seems necessary to cite evidence in support of the view that the psychological and social adjustment of people affected by SCD depends as much on these factors as on characteristics of the patient and the condition, and there is similarly little doubt that considerable scope for improvement exists in both the provision and the delivery of supportive services for SCD. One of the most striking features of the literature is the gulf between the recommendations of authorities in the field on appropriate levels and forms of care for SCD, and the reports of patients about the services they actually need and receive. Some of the biggest problems would appear to be in the area of service delivery, on which a very broad consensus exists over the best way to set about making improvements. Almost all of those who have considered the question, from leading authorities in centres of excellence for the care of SCD to voluntary organizations working on behalf of those affected, have advocated better integration and coordination of services at all stages, including assessment, planning, care, and follow-up, in order to make the best use of available resources, ensure that those in need do not slip through the healthcare net, and ensure that identified needs are met appropriately.

Individual needs assessment is probably the first requirement for the implementation of a truly 'psychosocial' approach to care for SCD. Assessment of this kind should recognize the interplay between aspects of education, family dynamics, and social and economic factors, as well as medical considerations, each of which should be taken into account when planning programmes of care for people affected by SCD.

A multidimensional view of the impact of chronic illness on everyday life has often been advocated on the basis of sociological analyses (Bury, 1991), and some have argued recently that the management of chronic illness should be placed within a more comprehensive 'systems' approach (Shute and Paton, 1992). Such an approach emphasizes the importance of bringing together medical, biological, psychological, and social factors in the assessment of patients, and of considering possible interactions between treatments and aspects of the person and their environment rather than viewing diseases in isolation (Schwartz, 1981). An important feature of such approaches is the key role they provide for psychology in the holistic assessment of patients as individuals, and the tailoring of treatment packages to meet individual needs. Psychology has so far played only a minor role in the care and support of people with SCD, but the discipline has a great deal of expertise and skills to offer. As Schwartz (1982) has pointed out: 'It should ultimately be the psychologists' responsibility to demonstrate the importance of the discipline's basic and clinical findings to the interdisciplinary field of behaviour medicine.'

The co-ordination and integration of existing services could achieve the most immediate and direct benefit to people affected by SCD, but it is not the only area in which measures could be

125

taken to improve the level and quality of care in SCD. Many authors (Pless and Perrin, 1985; Nash, 1986) have drawn attention to possible improvements in areas such as public education, outreach work, in-service training for health care professionals, research, and collaboration between statutory agencies and organizations in the voluntary sector, all of which would be expected to raise the profile of SCD generally and contribute to better prospects for people affected by SCD in the longer term. All such measures require a greater level of political and financial commitment, the absence of which could be viewed as the chief obstacle to the provision of improved systems of service and support for SCD, for most of the recommendations made about service provision in relation to SCD during the 1980s are equally relevant and valid in the 1990s.

Theoretical Integration

The development and application of theory is probably the area in which least progress has been made in our social and psychological understanding of SCD. Most of what we know comes from rather piecemeal studies of practically or clinically oriented aspects of the condition, and although some studies have incorporated a range of variables in multivariate analyses in attempts to develop models of coping (Moise, 1986), there have been few attempts to integrate findings into coherent theoretical models of health and illness. The value of theory for its own sake can be overstated, and elaborate, overarching models with little explanatory or predictive power contribute little either to our understanding of the problem or to the welfare of those directly affected. However, individual findings are difficult to build upon unless they can be cast in a wider conceptual framework, and good theoretical work serves to stimulate more thoughtful research, establishes links between findings in different areas, and can challenge established ways of thinking about illness and health.

The absence of more theoretical approaches in research on SCD is perhaps surprising because the development and application of theory has been an important feature of recent work in health psychology more generally. The health belief model, in which elements of a person's perception of the threat of illness and of the benefit to be obtained by adopting healthier practices are used to predict health-related behaviour (Rosenstock, 1966), has been applied to the practice of preventive medicine, compliance with medical advice, use of medical services, and a wide range of health-related behaviours, many of which are relevant to the management of SCD. Similarly, the theory of reasoned action, in which behavioural intentions are considered as the product of attitudes towards the behaviour in question and perceptions of normative values (Ajzen and Fishbein, 1980) has been used to examine smoking, family planning, drinking and drug use, and exercising and weight loss. Again, the scope for applying the theory to aspects of SCD such as the avoidance of sickling crises is considerable.

Stress is another area of relatively well developed theory with scope for application to coping and adjustment in SCD. In Selye's model (Selye, 1976), stress represents an abnormal response to environmental demands and is mediated by a number of factors, including the characteristics of the individual, the environment, the social support available, and the cultural background. Factors relating to stress have been shown to play a role in coping with SCD, but in contrast to other areas of health behaviour, where the effects of stress and stress management on health and health behaviour have been examined in more detail, the concept of stress has not been applied very widely in relation to SCD.

Future Research

Almost every aspect of the psychology of SCD deserves greater attention. There would, however, be little point in duplicating research that has already been conducted, or in extending the range of topics covered by limited and piecemeal studies. We attempt here to indicate worthwhile areas for future research and to identify the types of study that we believe would make the most useful advances in our understanding.

Subgroups within the Sickle Cell Disease Population

One of the most important reasons for inconclusive findings in many areas of research is the fact that people with SCD are not a homogenous population. The wide variability in adjustment and coping is now well established by studies with general samples of

127

people with SCD, and more progress in understanding the dynamics of problem areas and positive aspects of coping would be achieved by focusing on particular groups of affected people. The most important group in this respect is those who are most at risk of significant psychological and social problems as a direct or indirect result of SCD. Detailed studies of the factors that contribute to raised risk of maladjustment would enable the development of SCD-related psychological problems to be better understood in theoretical terms, and would assist in the design of more effective preventive and protective measures. A better understanding of the links between risk factors and the manifestation of psychosocial complications would also contribute to more reliable identification of those who would benefit most from supportive interventions.

Conversely, a better understanding of the factors and processes that contribute to positive aspects of coping and adjustment would be obtained by focusing on those who appear to be most resilient to the potential limitations and difficulties associated with SCD. The greatest need in this area is for practical measures that would enable coping skills and strategies to be adopted more widely, and the most valuable findings would be those that related more abstract factors associated with coping, such as perceived control, to everyday habits and behaviours in such a way that affected individuals and health care professionals could act directly on research findings to improve the quality of life of those affected by SCD.

A third group of people who have been relatively neglected by research in this area is older adults. There is a growing population of people with SCD who are living longer, and whose needs and problems have not been fully addressed. The literature on the way such individuals cope with problems in areas of employment, relationships, and parenthood is very limited, and more focused attention to the emerging needs of this group would be welcome. To some extent, however, our limited understanding of the problems faced by adults with SCD is due to the way that people of different age groups have been studied separately, with the result that the difficulties presented by SCD for people at different periods of their lives have been treated as separate phenomena. Coping and adjustment later in life might well be influenced by experiences and events during childhood or adolescence, but possible links between early and later adjustment would only be revealed by longitudinal studies, or research with a lifespan perspective, that would enable adjustment in different areas and at different periods of life to be more closely related within a developmental framework.

Pain Research

The phenomenon of pain has received considerable attention within both medicine and psychology, and the care of people affected by SCD could probably be improved by a more widespread and consistent application of existing knowledge and expertise in the management of pain. This is not to say that we do not need to know more about the most effective ways to control pain in SCD. Medical advances in our understanding of the sickling process would enable pain crises to be avoided and treated more effectively, and there is considerable scope for improvements in our understanding of the best ways to approach the management of pain for different groups of patients. Children are such a group, for as McGrath (1989, p. 361) has pointed out, 'Despite significant advances in our ability to control pain, the clinical management of children's pain is still deficient.'

Evidence about the experiences of patients with SCD pain, and about the views and practices of many medical staff, suggest that many people with SCD do not receive the best available clinical services in relation to pain management. Where there are such shortfalls in clinical service provision they would appear to be due, at least in part, to assumptions that people with SCD are at risk of dependence on drugs provided for the relief of pain. The best way to approach such a problem is to collect reliable evidence so that doctors would be better placed to make good clinical judgements about managing SCD pain, for hard facts on the scale of drug abuse and dependency among people with SCD are conspicuously lacking at present. The absence of reliable statistics on the subject may incline doctors to fall back on conservative prescribing practices, and to be influenced in some cases by stereotypical misconceptions about SCD pain and drug abuse.

Data is needed about the use of drugs of both medical and illegal origin by people with SCD as a function of clinical, personal, and social factors, in order to establish the true scale of undermedication and dependency associated with SCD, and to identify those who may be at risk of inappropriate pain management regimes. The quality of clinical service provision in relation to SCD pain could also be approached from the other side of the issue, by examining knowledge and attitudes about the management of

SCD pain among medical staff as a function of their experiences in this area, their practices and policies, and the experiences of their patients.

People with SCD would also benefit from improvements in the effectiveness of non-medical management of pain, for such methods have the potential to reduce their dependency on medical services. Various behavioural methods for the control of SCD pain have been examined in a rather limited way, but more controlled trials conducted over longer periods are needed before we could be confident of the benefits of such methods. Larger scale studies capable of taking individual differences into account would also be welcome, for the effectiveness of any behavioural strategy is likely to vary from person to person, and there is at present little evidence on which to base recommendations about how to match programmes to people for best results.

Many non-pharmacological methods for the control of pain, such as hypnosis, biofeedback, and acupuncture come from outside the Western medical tradition, but techniques with specific African origins have not, to our knowledge, been investigated in relation to SCD. The range of behavioural methods to be considered could therefore be extended to include those with a basis in the tradition of the culture concerned, and any study of pain management would benefit from taking account of distinct attitudes or beliefs about pain associated with the culture of the affected person.

Towards a Better Understanding of the Affected Population

The third area in which research is needed relates to almost every aspect of SCD. This need is for a better general understanding of the populations affected by SCD. Where a condition affects only certain groups within society, and those groups are underrepresented among those forming policy, providing care, and conducting research, there is considerable scope for progress to be impeded by misplaced assumptions and incomplete understanding about the behaviour, attitudes and values of the client group on the part of professionals. Difficulties could arise through the misinterpretation of findings, or through attempts to implement measures that run counter to established ways of thinking and behaving among those affected.

Any findings that relate the presence of SCD to the incidence of particular problems needs to take account of the outcome that might be expected in the absence of SCD, and in many cases this information is not readily available. For example, in order to make a realistic assessment of the impact of SCD on family life one must first understand the prevailing patterns of familial organization and dynamics among the population most affected by SCD. Rates of separation and divorce, the significance of extended families, or relations between parents and children observed in the presence of SCD are not interpretable unless they can be considered in a meaningful context, yet there is at present very little understanding among the mainstream medical and research professions about the distinctive features of family life and organization among ethnic minority communities. In other cases, what is lacking may be not so much facts about the demographics of the relevant population so much as a greater appreciation of the ways in which psychological responses to SCD could be influenced by cultural factors such as attitudes to heredity, illness, and disability. Either way, more ethnographic research on relevant aspects of the African, Afro-Caribbean and other affected communities would increase the power of psychological studies to provide meaningful insights into the social and psychological implications of SCD. Greater involvement by members of the affected communities among the professional groups concerned would also, of course, reduce the scope for problems of this kind.

Factors like these are also important in the application of findings, for measures based on invalid assumptions about the client group are less likely to be effective than those that are tailored to take account of relevant preferences, attitudes, or needs of those intended to benefit. There is a great deal of work to be done to develop better methods for the assessment of the needs of affected families and individuals, for the matching of services to needs, for the training of staff, and for the evaluation of services. Again, the quality of care for SCD could also be improved by drawing directly on the knowledge and skills of individuals from the same ethnic groups as those affected by SCD.

Sickle Cell Disease in a Wider Context

This is not a political book. Rather, we have attempted to present the clearest possible picture of the social and psychological implications of SCD from the perspective of the social scientist, based on an assessment of the available empirical evidence. However, there is a political dimension to SCD that no comprehensive analysis can exclude. The politics of SCD relate mainly to the social and economic status of the ethnic groups most affected by the condition in the Western world, who are disadvantaged in a range of ways, including the provision of, and access to, health care.

Much of the research we have reviewed here has drawn attention, directly or indirectly, to social and economic aspects of the problems related to SCD. Many of the difficulties encountered originate in, or are compounded by, social or economic disadvantages, which would place those affected at greater risk of poor physical and psychological health even in the absence of SCD. Black people have lower incomes on average than white people (Oppenheim, 1990), and are exposed to poorer housing conditions (Phillips, 1987). Minimum standards of living conditions are preconditions for the achievement of an acceptable quality of life, and disadvantages in areas like income and housing are major obstacles to effective coping with chronic illness. It is no surprise, therefore, that factors related to social or economic status are among the most reliable correlates of adjustment in samples of people with SCD.

The inequalities affecting the groups to which SCD is mainly confined also extend to the quality of health care they receive. Analyses of ethnicity and health (Torkington, 1991) have concluded that black people get a poorer deal than whites in almost every respect. Current service provision for SCD lacks a cohesive and well formulated model for psychosocial assessment and intervention, and the needs of those affected by SCD have been generally neglected. Where policy and planning has addressed the problems posed by SCD, guidelines and recommendations have not been matched by the experiences and perceptions of those who are intended to benefit. Similar, and legitimate, critiques of service provision can be made on behalf of those affected by many other conditions. In relation to chronic illnesses of childhood, for example, Eiser (1990b) has suggested that:

> The psychological needs of any single disease group may be under-estimated or dismissed, because they are too small to be an effective lobby. This may be of practical significance, when it comes to pressing for resources at home or school – it may be more persuasive to demand additional resources for all chronically sick children and their families than isolated cases.

132

This is probably true of conditions for which there is not also an ethnic dimension, but the convergence of factors placing those affected by SCD at multiple disadvantage means that to bracket SCD with other chronic illnesses would understate the need for improvements in service provision. In any case, levels of funding for research and support for comparable chronic illnesses are already far better developed than for SCD. Black and Laws (1986) have made the point that cystic fibrosis attracts around 40 times more financial support than SCD, although both affect similar numbers of people. Hurtig and Viera (1986) have suggested that racial and cultural factors have contributed to the relative neglect of SCD in many areas of health care.

A good deal is already known about SCD and its management, and significant improvements in the prospects of those affected could be achieved simply by applying existing expertise. The implementation of scientific advances have often been influenced by factors such as changes in the law, the economy, or public awareness, and it seems likely that a significant shift in attitudes and priorities will be needed before sufferers of SCD begin to feel the full benefit of what is already known about the condition.

Racism permeates thinking and practice in many areas, including science, medicine, and law. Konotey-Ahulu (1991) has detailed a catalogue of extraordinary medical and scientific publications in which sickle cell trait has been confused with SCD, with the effect of grossly exaggerating the (minimal) risk of illness associated with the trait. Misleading public statements of this kind have contributed to significant discrimination against trait carriers in employment, in obtaining life and health care insurance, and in legislation. Bowman (1975), for example, has described how legislation in the United States on mandatory screening for genetic diseases has unfairly penalized those with SCD or the sickle cell trait, and there is evidence (Konotey-Ahulu, 1991) that much medical and social practice in relation to SCD has conformed to an invisible philosophy that holds that elimination of the genes responsible for SCD is a more desirable objective than support for affected individuals. Whitten and Fischhoff (1974) have drawn attention to the misleading and alarmist way in which SCD has been described in many scientific and lay accounts of the condition. Misinformed television programmes and magazine articles have compounded the problems faced by people with SCD by creating anxiety in those directly affected by the condition and contributing to prejudicial attitudes and opinions among the general public.

133

Many of the worst excesses of this kind have taken place in the United States, where awareness of SCD and the provision of care has since improved significantly – many of the best-developed and most enlightened programmes for the support of those affected by SCD are now to be found in that country. The point, however, is that where a medical condition is confined mainly to particular ethnic groups, the potential will always exist for the provision of care to be affected by punitive racial or cultural considerations. There are no grounds for complacency in this area for there is still a good deal to be done in the improvement of care for SCD, and while those social groups who are most affected by the condition remain significantly disadvantaged in almost every other important way, it is virtually inevitable that the scale and quality of services for SCD will fall below optimal levels.

Considering the importance of social, economic, and political factors in the welfare of people affected by SCD, one might take the view that the potential contribution of psychology is at best limited and at worst trivial or even diversionary. Certainly, attention to psychological aspects of the condition should not distract from the need for improvements in more basic social and economic aspects of the circumstances of those affected. A more equal society is desirable from the point of view of individual and public health, and a radical appraisal of the nature and scale of the health care problem presented by SCD would probably attach a low priority to psychological measures, but psychology has a role to play in promoting fairer treatment for those affected by SCD as well as in the development of specific psychological interventions. Many psychological studies have highlighted the social and economic factors that influence psychological adjustment and well-being, and many of the more basic shortfalls in service provision are related to underlying attitudes and beliefs, which fall directly within the scope of psychology.

Work in this area requires the adoption of a wide perspective, for SCD is a multifaceted health care problem. Progress in any single area is likely to have less overall impact than more gradual and general improvements over a range of areas, including medicine, social services, legislation, and public opinion. Psychological factors may appear trivial when compared with the social and economic dimensions of the problem, but a greater understanding of the psychological elements of the situation can help to facilitate changes in other areas by addressing underlying misconceptions, ignorance, and unhelpful attitudes, as well as by assisting in the co-ordination and integration of other services.

Glossary

Acidosis: A condition in which the blood is abnormally acid.

Alleles: One of two or more alternative forms of a gene.

Amino acids: An organic compound of 20 chemicals containing an amino group ($-NH_2$) and a carboxyl group ($-COOH$), they are constituents of all proteins.

Amniocentesis: Withdrawal of the liquid surrounding the fetus in the mother's womb for testing.

Anaemia: The condition caused by a reduced level of haemoglobin in the blood.

Analgesia: Drugs for relief of pain.

Antenatal: (Meaning before birth). Concerned with the care and treatment of the unborn child and of pregnant women.

AS: Sickle cell trait (cannot develop into sickle cell disease). AS individuals are healthy carriers.

Arthralgia: Pain in one or more joints.

Asplenia: Absence of the normal functions of the spleen. Common in sickle cell anaemia. Results in an increased risk of bacterial infections.

Bilirubin: A red bile pigment formed from haemoglobin during the destruction of erythrocytes.

Bone marrow: Tissue of the internal cavities of the bones, where new red and white blood cells develop.

Carcinogenic: Producing or tending to produce cancer.

Chromosomes: Bodies in the cell nucleus that are the bearers of genes. There are 46 (23 pairs) in almost every human cell.

Chronic illness: Medical condition that affects individuals for extended periods of time, often for life. Generally, chronic illnesses cannot be cured.

CNS: Central nervous system, includes the brain and the spinal cord, responsible for the integration of all nervous activities.

Control group: A group in a study that is as closely matched as possible (e.g. sex, age, ethnic origin, etc.) to the group of patients under investigation.

Dactylitis: Inflammation of the bones of the hands or feet.

DNA: (Deoxyribonucleic Acid). A large molecule found principally in the chromosomes of the cell nucleus. Genetic information is coded in the sequence of molecular subunits (bases) that are the constituents of the molecule.

Dominant gene: A gene capable of making its effect apparent regardless of whether the allele is the same or different.

Eclampsia: A serious condition affecting women towards the end of pregnancy, causing convulsions and coma.

Electromyogram (EMG): The technique of recording the electrical activity of a muscle, used to assess nerve and muscle problems.

Electrophoresis: A technique used in blood analysis to detect sickle cell disease and other abnormal haemoglobins.

Erythrocytes: Red blood cells containing the protein haemoglobin that carries oxygen.

Femur: The proximal bone of the hind or lower limb. In humans it is the longest and largest bone, extending from the hip to the knee.

Fetal haemoglobin (HbF): A haemoglobin variant that predominates in the blood of a newborn and persists in some forms of anaemia.

Gene: The functional unit of heredity which occupies a specific location on a chromosome and consists of a specific sequence of bases in DNA. A gene is capable of reproducing itself exactly at each cell division, and of directing the formation of an enzyme or other protein.

Globin: A protein chain that forms part of a haemoglobin molecule.

Haematopoietic stem cells: Cells in the bone marrow involved in the formation of blood cells in the living body.

Haemoglobin: An iron-containing protein pigment occuring in the blood cells of vertebrates and functioning primarily in the transport of oxygen from the lungs to the tissues of the body.

Haemolysis: Dissolution of red blood cells with liberation of oxygen.

HbF: Fetal haemoglobin.

Heterozygous: The condition in which members of a pair of genes determining a particular characteristic are dissimilar.

Homogenous: Of uniform structure or composition throughout.

Homozygous: The condition in which members of pair of genes are identical.

Humerus: The longest bone of the upper arm extending from the shoulder to the elbow.

Hydrophobic: Having a propensity to repel water.

136

Hydroxyurea: An antineoplastic drug used to treat some forms of leukaemia.

Hypoventilation: Abnormally shallow or slow breathing, which can cause low levels of oxygen in the blood.

Hypoxaemia: A deficient oxygenation of the blood.

Hypoxia: A deficiency of oxygen reaching the tissues of the body.

In vitro (in glass): Outside the living body and in an artificial environment.

IQ: (Intelligence Quotient). Level of intelligence as compared to the population average.

Jaundice: A yellow appearance of the eyes and skin indicating excess bilirubin in the blood.

Locus of control: A term in social psychology used to refer to the perceived source of control (internal or external) over one's behaviour.

Malaria: An infectious disease characterized by high fever, caused by the presence of a parasite in the red blood cells. Transmitted by mosquito bites.

Meiosis: A type of cell division that produces four cells, each having half the number of chromosomes of the original cell.

Menarche: Onset of menstruation.

Microfilament: The minute protein filaments that are widely distributed in the cytoplasm of cells and which help to maintain their structural framework and play a role in the movement of cell components.

Molecule: Smallest unit of a substance capable of existing independently.

Opiate: A group of drugs derived from opium, including codeine, papaverine, morphine, heroin, and pethidine.

Osteoporosis: A condition characterized by decrease in bone mass with decreasing density and enlargement of bone spaces.

Pain crises: The most common problem in SCD; see *vaso-occlusive crises*.

Parenteral: Situated or occuring outside the intestine, or introduced otherwise than by way of the intestine.

Pathognomonic: Distinctively characteristic of a particular disease or condition.

pH: A measure of the acidity or alkalinity of a solution (e.g. blood).

Phenotype: The visible characteristics of an organism that are produced by the interaction of the genotype and the environment.

Placebo: A pill or medicine without any pharmacological effect, used in studies testing new drugs to separate pharmacological from psychological effects.

Platelet: A disc-shaped particle present in the peripheral blood, needed to arrest bleeding.

Pneumococcal infection: Serious bacterial infection, often pneumonia.

Polymerisation: Chemical reaction in which two or more small molecules combine to form larger molecules that contain repeating structural units of the original molecules.

Prenatal: Relating to or occuring in the period before birth.

prn: As needed, or as the circumstances require, used in writing prescriptions.

Prodromal: Earliest stage of an illness or pain crises in SCD, it relates to the period of time before the first physical symptoms and the onset of pain.

Prophylactic: Treatment or measure that prevents or helps to prevent disease.

Protein: One of a group of compounds made up of one or more chains of amino acids, they are constituents of the body.

Psychopathology: The scientific study of mental disorders.

Psychosocial: A term used to describe any situation where both psychological and social factors are assumed to play a role.

Recessive gene: A member of a pair of genes whose effect is not apparent in the presence of its more dominant allele.

SβThal: Sickle β Thalassaemia. Results from the pairing of the sickle cell gene and βThalassaemia gene.

SC: SC disease. Results from the combination of the sickle cell and haemoglobin C genes, generally a mild form of sickle cell disease.

SCD: Sickle cell disease. The family of blood disorders including sickle cell anaemia, SC disease, and sickle β Thalassaemia.

Sickled cell: A damaged red blood cell distorted into a characteristic crescent or sickle shape.

Spleen: Abdominal organ closely associated with the circulatory system. It plays a role in the maintenance of blood volume, the production of some types of blood cell, and the recovery of material from worn out red cells.

Splenic sequestration: A serious situation in which red blood cells collect in the spleen.

SS: Sickle cell anaemia: The most severe form of sickle cell disease.

Steady state: Periods of time during which patients feel well and do not experience painful crises.

Teratogenic: Relating to or causing developmental abnormalities.

Thalassaemia: Hereditary blood disease in which there is a reduction in globin chain production due to an abnormal thalassaemia globin gene.

Trait: A characteristic of healthy carriers of recessive genes responsible for an illness, e.g. sickle cell trait; *see* **AS**.

Vaso-occlusive crises: Commonly known as pain crises. Caused by the obstruction of blood flow. These are the main symptoms of sickle cell disease.

Sickle Cell and Thalassaemia Centres in the UK

Centres in London

BRENT
Sickle Cell and Thalassaemia
Centre
Central Middlesex Hospital
Acton Lane
London NW10 7NS
Tel: 081 453–2262

CROYDON
12–18 Leonard Road
Croydon Surrey CR9 2RS
Tel: 081 680–2008 extension
292

EALING
Specialist Nurse SCD/Thal
Mattock Lane Health Centre
Ealing
London W13 9NS
Tel: 081 574–2444 extension
2933

GREENWICH
Sickle and Thalassaemia
Centre
Market Street Health Centre
Market Street
London SE18 6QR
Tel: 081 858–5427

ISLINGTON
Sickle and Thalassaemia
Centre
Royal Northern Hospital
Holloway Road
London N7 6LD
Tel: 071 272–7777 extension
351

NEWHAM
Sickle and Thalassaemia
Centre
Plaistow Hospital
Samson Street
London E13 9EH
Tel: 081 472–3011

CITY AND HACKNEY
St Leonards Hospital
Nuttal Street
London N1 5LZ
Tel: 071 601–7762

St Bartholomew's Hospital
Department of Haematology
West Smithfield
London EC1A 7BE
Tel: 071 601–8051

HARINGEY
The George Marsh Sickle and
Thalassaemia Centre
St. Ann's Hospital
St. Ann's Road
London N15 3TH
Tel: 081 809–1797

LAMBETH
Sickle and Thalassaemia
Centre
2 Stockwell Mews
London SW9 9EN
Tel: 071 737–3588

ST THOMAS'S HOSPITAL
c/o Community Midwives
Haydon Ward
St. Thomas's Hospital
London SE1 7EH
Tel: 071 928–9292 extension
3123

WALTHAM FOREST
Sickle and Thalassaemia
Centre
Leyton Green Clinic
Leyton Green Road
London E10 6BL
Tel: 081 539–8646

Centres outside London

BIRMINGHAM
Sickle and Thalassaemia
Centre
Ladywood Health Centre
395 Ladywood Middleway
Ladywood
Birmingham B1 2TP
Tel: 021 454–4262

LIVERPOOL
Sickle and Thalassaemia
Centre
Abercromby Health Centre
Groove Street
Liverpool L7 7HG
Tel: 051 708–9370

CARDIFF
Sickle and Thalassaemia
Centre
Butetown Health Centre
Loudoun Square
Docks
Cardiff CF1 5UZ
Tel: 0222 488026

LEEDS
Sickle and Thalassaemia
Centre
Chapeltown Health Centre
Spencer Place
Leeds LS7 4BB
Tel: 0532 485522

BRISTOL
Sickle and Thalassaemia
Centre
90 Lower Cheltenham Place
Montpelier
Bristol BS6 5LE
Tel: 0272 411880

The Lodge
31 Tyndalls Park Road
Bristol BS8 1PH
Tel: 0272 741419

DERBY (SOUTH)
Sickle and Thalassaemia
Centre
Pear Tree Clinic
Pear Tree Road
Derby DE3 6QD
Tel: 0332 254770

MANCHESTER
Sickle and Thalassaemia
Centre
Moss Side Health Centre
Monton Street
Manchester M14 4PG
Tel: 061 226–8972 extension
213/214

NOTTINGHAM
Sickle and Thalassaemia
Centre
Victoria Health Centre
Glass House Street
Nottingham NG1 3LW
Tel: 0602 480500

WOLVERHAMPTON
Sickle and Thalassaemia
Centre
The Advent Community
Church Hall
Himley Crescent
Goldhorn Park
Wolverhampton WV4 5DE
Tel: 0902 331161

READING
c/o Haematology Department
Royal Berkshire Hospital
Craven Road
Berkshire RG1 5AN
Tel: 0734 877689

National Voluntary Organizations for Sickle Cell and Thalassaemia

**Organization for Sickle Cell
Anaemia Research (OSCAR)**
Sickle Cell Community Centre
Tiverton Road
Tottenham
London N15 6RT
Tel: 081 802–3055/0944

**Sickle Cell Anaemia Relief
(SCAR)**
4 Palmerston Court
Palmerston Way
London SW8 4DA
Tel: 071 720–2076

Sickle Cell Society
54 Station Road
Harlesden
London NW10 4UB
Tel: 081 961–7795/4006

UK Thalassaemia Society
107 Nightingale Lane
London N8 7QY
Tel: 081 348–0437

Comprehensive Sickle Cell Centres in the USA

ALABAMA
University of South Alabama
College of Medicine
Dept. of Pediatrics
1504 Spring Hill Avenue
Mobile, AL 36340
Tel: (205) 434–3915
Director: Rob Skeel

CALIFORNIA
University of Southern California
Raulston Medical Research 306
2025 Zonal Avenue
Los Angeles, CA 90033
Tel: (213) 342–1259
Director: Page Johnson

San Francisco General Hospital
1001 Porero Avenue,
Room 6J-5
San Francisco, CA 94110
Tel: (415) 206–5169
Director: William C. Mentzer

GEORGIA
Georgia-N.I.H. CSCC
Grady Health System
80 Butler Street, S.E.
P.O. Box 26109
Atlanta, GA 30335
Tel: (404) 616–3572
Director: James Eckman

MASSACHUSETTS
Boston City Hospital
818 Harrison Avenue FGH-2
Boston, MA 02118
Tel: (617) 534–5727
Director: Lillian E.C. McMahon

NEW YORK
Montefiore Hospital Medical
Center
111 E. 210th Street
Bronx, NY 10467
Tel: (718) 920–7373/7375
Director: Ronald L. Nagel
Clinical Dir.: Lennette J.
Benjamin

College of Physicians and
Surgeons
Columbia University
630 West 168th Street
New York, NY 10032
Tel: (212) 305–5808
Director: Sergio Piomelli

NORTH CAROLINA
Duke University Medical Center
Durham, NC 27710
Tel: (919) 684–6464
Co-Director: Wendell Rosse, and
Thomas R. Kinney

PENNSYLVANIA
Children's Hospital of
Philadelphia
34th Street & Civic Center
Boulevard
Philadelphia, PA 19104
Tel: (215) 590–3423
Director: Kwaku
Ohene-Frempong

TENNESSEE
Meharry Medical College
1005 D.B. Todd Junior Boulevard
Nashville, TN 37208
Tel: (615) 327–6763
Director: Ernest A. Turner

References

Abrams, S.J. (1987). The self concept of sickle cell children and their siblings and related maternal attitudes. *Dissertation Abstracts International*, **47**, 3869-A.

Adekile, A.D., Adeodu, O.O., Fadulu, S.O., Weinhemer, A., and Sanduja, D. (1990). Preliminary clinical trial of Nix-06999 in the management of sickle cell anaemia. *Nigerian Medical Journal*, **20**, 1.

Ajzen, I. and Fishbein, M. (1980). *Understanding attitudes and predicting social behaviour*. Englewood Cliffs, NY: Prentice-Hall.

Akenzua, G.I. (1990). Screening for psychosocial dysfunction in children with sickle cell anaemia. *Nigerian Journal of Paediatrics*, **17** (1&2), 15–21.

Alleyne, S.I., Wint, E., and Serjeant, G.R. (1977). Social effects of leg ulceration in sickle cell anemia. *Southern Medical Journal*, **70**, 213–214.

Anderson, H.R., Bailey, P.A., Cooper, J.A., Palmer, J.S., and West, S. (1983). Morbidity and school absence caused by asthma and wheezing illness. *Archives of Diseases in Childhood*, **58**, 777–784.

Anionwu, E. (1977). Self-help in sickle cell anaemia. *World Medicine*, **12**, 89–91.

Anionwu, E. (1983). Sickle cell disease: Screening and counselling in the antenatal and neonatal period – Part 1. *Midwife, Health Visitor and Community Nurse*, **19**, 402–406.

Anionwu, E. (1989a). Sickle cell anaemia. *African Woman*, **2**(4), 13–15.

Anionwu, E. (1989b). Running a sickle cell centre: Community counselling. In J.K. Cruickshank and D. Beevers (Eds), *Ethnic factors in health and disease*. London: Wright.

Anionwu, E. (1992). Sickle cell disorders and the schoolchild. *Health Visitor*, **65**, 120–122.

Anionwu, E. and Beattie, A. (1981). Learning to cope with SCD. A parent's experience. *Nursing Times*, **July 8th**, 1214–1220.

Aschenbrenner, J. (1975). *Lifelines: Black families in Chicago*. New York: Holt, Rinehart and Winston.

Atkin, K. and Rollings, J. (1992). Informal care in Asian and Afro/ Caribbean communities: A literature review. *British Journal of Social Work*, **22**, 405–418.

Bainbridge, R., Higgs, D.R., Maude, G.H., and Serjeant, G.R. (1985). Clinical presentation of homozygous sickle cell disease. *Journal of Pediatrics*, **106**, 881–885.

Bamisaiye, A., Bakare, C.R., and Olatawura, M.O. (1974). Some social-psychological dimensions of sickle cell anemia amongst Nigerians. *Clinical Pediatrics*, **13** (1), 56–59.

Barnhart, M.I., Henry, R.L., and Lusher, J.M. (1976). *Sickle/Cell*. Kalamazoo, MI: A scope publication, The Upjohn Company.

Bell, J. (1991). Pain and addiction. *Drug and Alcohol Review*, **10**, 247–252.

Bertram, R.A., Webster, G.D., and Carson, C.C. (1985). Priapism: Aetiology, treatment, and results in series of thirty five presentations. *Urology*, **26**, 229–231.

Bianco, I., Graziano, B., Lerone, M., Congedo, P., Ponzini, D., Braconi, F., and Aliquo, C. (1984). A screening programme for the prospective prevention of Mediterranean anaemia in Latium: Results of seven years' work. *Journal of Medical Genetics*, **21**, 268–271.

Black, J. and Laws, S. (1986). *Living with SCD. An enquiry into the need for health and social service provision for sickle cell sufferers in Newham*. London: East London Sickle Cell Society.

Bowman, J.E. (1975). Ethical, legal, and humanistic implications of sickle cell programs. *INSERM*, **44**, 353–378.

Breslau, N., Weitzman, M., and Messenger, K. (1981). Psychologic functioning of siblings of disabled children. *Pediatrics*, **67** (3), 344–353.

Broadhead, W.E., Kaplan, O.O., Sherman, A.J., Wagner, E.H., Schoenback, V.J., Grimson, R., Hayden, G.T., and Gehlback, S.N. (1983). The epidemiologic evidence for a relationship between social support and health. *Journal of Epidemiology*, **117**, 521–537.

Brookoff, D. (1991). Treating the patient in pain. *Emergency Medicine*, **May 30th**, 58–69.

Brookoff, D. (1992). A protocol for defusing sickle cell crisis. *Emergency Medicine*, **January 15th**, 131–140.

Broome, M. and Monroe, S. (1979). *Sickle cell anemia: A patient-perceived needs assessment*. San Francisco, CA: Sickle Cell Anemia Research and Education, Inc.

Brown, C. (1984). *Black and white Britain: The third PSI survey*. London: Heinemann.

Brozovic, M. and Anionwu, E. (1984). Sickle cell disease in Britain. *Journal of Clinical Pathology*, **37**, 1321–1326.

Brozovic, M. and Davies, S.C. (1987). Management of sickle cell disease. *Postgraduate Medical Journal*, **63**; 605–609.

Brozovic, M., Davies, S.C., Yardumian, A., Bellingham, A., Marsh, G., and Stephens, A.D. (1986). Pain relief in sickle cell crises. *Lancet*, **September 13th**, 624–625.

Brozovic, M., Davies, S.C., and Brownell, A.I. (1987). Acute admissions of patients with sickle cell disease who live in Britain. *British Medical Journal*, **294**, 1206–1208.

Brozovic, M., Davies, S.C., and Henthorn, J. (1989). Haematological and clinical aspects of sickle cell disease in Britain. In J.K. Cruickshank and D. Beevers, (Eds), *Ethnic factors in health and disease*. London: Wright.

147

Burlew, A.K., Evans, R., and Oler, C. (1989). The impact of a child with sickle cell disease on family dynamics. *Annals of the New York Academy of Sciences*, **565**, 161–171.

Burr, C.K. (1985). Impact on the family of a chronically ill child. In N. Hobbs and J.M. Perrin (Eds), *Issues in the care of children with chronic illness*. San Francisco CA: Jossey-Bass.

Bury, M. (1991). The sociology of chronic illness: A review of research and prospects. *Sociology of Health and Illness*, **13**, 451–468.

Cadman, D. (1987). *Siblings: Similarities and differences. Findings of the Ontario Child Health Study*. Contemporary Issues in Child Psychiatry and Developmental Pediatrics Conference, Chedoke-McMaster Hospitals.

Cadman, D., Rosenbaum, P., Boyle, M., and Offord, D.R. (1991). Children with chronic illness: Family and parent demographic characteristics and psychosocial adjustment. *Pediatrics*, **87** (6), 884–889.

Cameron, B.F., Christian, E., Lobel, J.D., and Gaston, M.H. (1983). Evaluation of clinical severity in sickle cell disease. *Journal of the National Medical Association*, **75**, 483–487.

Cappelli, M., McGrath, P.J., MacDonald, N.E., Katsanis, J., and Lascelles, M. (1989). Parental care and overprotection of children with cystic fibrosis. *British Journal of Medical Psychology*, **62**, 281–289.

Charache, S. and Davies, S.C. (1991). Teaching both the management and the molecular biology of sickle cell disease. *Academic Medicine*, **66** (12), 48–49.

Charache, S., Lubin, B., and Reid, C.D. (1984). *Management and therapy of sickle cell disease*. Bethesda, MD: NIH Publications.

Chernoff, A., Shapleigh, J., and Moore, C. (1954). Therapy of chronic ulceration of legs associated with sickle cell anemia. *Journal of the American Medical Association*, **155**, 1487–1491.

Chodorkoff, J. and Whitten, C.F. (1963). Intellectual status of children with sickle cell anemia. *Journal of Pediatrics*, **63**, 29–35.

Cleeland, C.S. (1984). The impact of pain on the patient with cancer. *Cancer*, **54**, 2635–2641.

Cohen, S. and Syme, S.L. (1985) *Social support and health*. New York: Academic Press.

Collins, R. (1986). Psychological variables and interventions with patient population. In A.L. Hurtig and C.T. Viera (Eds), *Sickle cell disease: Psychological and psychosocial issues* (pp.62–74). Urbana, IL: University of Illinois.

Conley, C.L. (1980) Sickle-cell anemia – the first molecular disease. In M. Wintrobe (Ed), *Blood, pure and eloquent* (pp. 319–71). New York: McGraw-Hill.

Conyard, S., Krishnamurthy, M., and Dosik, H. (1980). Psychosocial aspects of sickle cell anemia in adolescents. *Health and Social Work* **5**(1), 20–26.

Cozzi, L., Tryon, W.W., and Sedlacek, K. (1987). The effectiveness of biofeedback-assisted relaxation in modifying sickle cell crises. *Biofeedback and Self-Regulation*, **12**, 51–61.

Crawford, M. (1991). Sickle cell disease in children. *Nursing*, **4**, 23–25.

Cummins, D., Heuschkel, R., and Davies, S.C. (1991). Penicillin prophylaxis in children with sickle cell disease in Brent. *British Medical Journal*, **302**, 989–990.

Dahl, J., Joranson, D., Engber, D., and Dosch, J. (1988). The cancer pain problem: Wisconsin's response. A report on the Wisconsin Cancer Pain Initiative. *Journal of Pain Symptom Management*, **3**, 1–20.

Damlouji, N.F., Kevess-Cohen, R., Charache, S., Georgopoulos, A., and Folstein, M.F. (1982). Social disability and psychiatric morbidity in sickle cell anaemia and diabetic patients. *Psychosomatics*, **23**, 925–931.

Daniels, D. (1990). Sickle cell anaemia: A patient's tale. *British Medical Journal*, **301**, 673.

Daniels, D., Moos, R.H., Billings, A.G., and Miller, J.J. (1987). Psychosocial risk and resistance factors among children with chronic illness, healthy siblings, and healthy controls. *Journal of Abnormal Child Psychology*, **15**, 295–308.

Davis, J.R., Vichinsky, E., and Lubin, B.H. (1980). Current treatment of sickle cell disease. *Current Problems in Pediatrics*, **10** (12), 1–64.

Davies, S.C. (1988a). Haemoglobinopathies – Where next? THS, **October**, 20.

Davies, S.C. (1988b). Obstetric implications of sickle cell disease. *Midwife, Health Visitor and Community Nurse*, **24**, 361–363.

Davies, S.C. (1993). Bone marrow transplant for sickle cell disease: The dilemma. *Blood Reviews*, **7**, 4–9.

Davies, S.C. and Brozovic, M. (1989). The presentation, management and prophylaxis of sickle cell disease. *Blood Reviews*, **3**, 30–44.

De Ceular, K., Gruber, C., Hayes, R. and Serjeant, G.R. (1982). Medroxyprogesterone acetate and homozygous SCD. *Lancet*, **ii**, 229–231.

Drotar, D. and Crawford, P. (1985). Psychological adaptation of siblings of chronically ill children: Research and practice implications. *Developmental and Behavioural Pediatrics*, **6**, 355–362.

Eiser, C. (1985). *The psychology of childhood illness*. New York: Springer-Verlag.

Eiser, C. (1990a). *Chronic childhood disease: An introduction to psychological theory and research*. Cambridge: Cambridge University Press.

Eiser, C. (1990b). Psychological effect of chronic disease. *Journal of Child Psychology and Psychiatry*, **31** (1), 85–98.

Elliot, C.H. and Olson, R.A. (1983). The management of children's distress in response to painful medical treatment for burn injuries. *Behaviour Research and Therapy*, **21**, 675–683.

Emery, A.E.H. and Pullen, I. (1984). *Psychological aspects of genetic counselling*. London: Academic Press.

Evans, R.C., Burlew, A.K., and Oler, C. (1988). Children with sickle cell anaemia: Parental relations, parent – child relations, and child behaviour. *Social Work*, **33** (2), 127–130.

Fenton, S. (1987). *Ageing minorities: Black people as they grow older in Britain*. London: Commission for Racial Equality.

Ferguson, M. (1991). Sickle cell anaemia and its effect on the new parent. *Health Visitor*, **64**, 73–76.

Ferrari, M. (1984). Chronic illness: Psychosocial effects on siblings-I. Chronically ill boys. *Journal of Child Psychology and Psychiatry*, **25** (3), 459–476.

Flanagan, C. (1980). Home management of sickle cell anemia. *Pediatric Nursing*, **6**, A–D.

Fordyce, W.E. (1976). *Behavioural methods for chronic pain and illness*. St Louis: C.V. Mosby Co.

Foster, S. (1991). My GP knows nothing about SCD. *General Practitioner*, **June 21st**, 40.

Fowler, M.C., Johnson, M.P., and Atkinson, S.S. (1985). School achievement and absence in children with chronic health conditions. *The Journal of Pediatrics*, **106**, 683–687.

Fowler, M.G., Whitt, J.K., Redding-Lallinger, R., Wells, R.J., Nash, K.B., and McMillan, C. (1986). Neuropsychologic deficits among school-age children with sickle cell disease. *American Journal of Diseases of Childhood*, **140**, 297.

France, R.D., Urban, B.J., and Keefe, F.J. (1984). Long-term use of narcotic analgesics in chronic pain. *Social Science and Medicine*, **19**, 1379–1382.

France-Dawson, M. (1990). Sickle cell conditions and health knowledge. *Nursing Standard*, **4**, 30–34.

Franklin, I.M. (1990). *Sickle Cell Disease: A Guide for Patients, Carers, and Health Workers*. London: Faber and Faber.

Franklin, I.M. and Atkin, K. (1986). Employment of persons with sickle cell disease and sickle cell trait. *Journal of the Society of Occupational Medicine*, **36** (3), 76–79.

Gaston, M. (1973). Management of children with sickle cell anaemia between crises. *Urban Health*, **2**, 24–26.

Gil, K.M., Abrams, M.R., Phillips, G., and Keefe, F.J. (1989). Sickle cell disease pain: Relation of coping strategies to adjustment. *Journal of Consulting and Clinical Psychology*, **57**, 725–731.

Gil, K.M., Williams, D.A., Thompson, Jr., R.J., and Kinney, T.R. (1991). Sickle cell disease in children and adolescents: The relation of child and parent pain coping strategies to adjustment. *Journal of Pediatric Psychology*, **16**, 643–663.

Gilbert, L. (1970). Intellectual impairment in children with sickle cell disease. *Dissertation Abstracts International*, **39**, 147B.

Gildenberg, P.L. and De Vaul, R.A. (1985). The chronic pain patient: Evaluation and management. *Pain and Headache*, **7**, 1–48.

Gonzalez, S., Steinglass, P., and Reiss, D. (1989). Putting the illness in its place: Discussion groups for families with chronic medical illnesses. *Family Process*, **28**, 69–87.

Graham, A.V., Reed, K.G., Levitt, C., Fine, M., and Medalie, J.H. (1982). Care of a troubled family and their child with sickle cell anaemia. *Journal of Family Practice*, **15**, 23–32.

Grath, A. (1977). Impact of abnormal child on parents. *British Journal of Psychiatry*, **130**, 405–410.

Gray, A., Anionwu, E., Davies, S.C., and Brozovic, M. (1991). Patterns of mortality in sickle cell disease in the United Kingdom. *Journal of Clinical Pathology*, **44** (6), 459–463.

152

Grossman, F.K. (1972). *Brothers and sisters of retarded children.* Syracuse, NY: Syracuse University Press.

Haertzen, C.A. and Hooks, M.T. (1969). Changes in personality and subjective experience associated with the chronic administration and withdrawal of opiates. *Journal of Nervous and Mental Diseases,* **148**, 606–614.

Hamre, M.R., Harmon, E.P., Kirkpatrick, D.V., Stern, M.J., and Humbert, J.R. (1991). Priapism as a complication of sickle cell disease. *Journal of Urology,* **145**, 1–5.

Hauri, D., Spycher, M., and Bruhlmann, W. (1983). Erection and priapism: A new physiopathological concept. *Urology International,* **38**, 138–140.

Herrick, J.B. (1910). Peculiar elongated and sickle-shaped red blood corpuscles in a case of severe anaemia. *Archives of Internal Medicine,* **6**, 517–521.

Hobbs, N., Perrin, J.M., and Ireys, H.T. (1985). *Chronically ill children and their families.* San Francisco: Jossey-Bass Publishers.

Hodenpyl, E. (1898). A case of apparent absence of the spleen, with general compensatory lymphatic hyperplasia. *Medical Record,* **54**, 695–698.

Holbrook, T. (1990). Patient-controlled analgesia pain management for children with sickle cell disease. *Journal of the Association for Academic Minority Physicians,* **1**, 93–96.

Horton, J.A.B. (1874). *The diseases of tropical climates and their treatment.* London: Churchill Livingstone.

Hurtig, A.L. (1986). The 'invisible' chronic illness in adolescence. In A.L. Hurtig and C.T. Viera (Eds), *Sickle cell disease: Psychological and psychosocial issues* (pp. 41–61). Urbana, IL: University of Illinois Press.

Hurtig, A.L. and Park, K.B. (1989). Adjustment and coping in adolescents with sickle cell disease. *Annals of the New York Academy of Sciences,* **565**, 172–182.

Hurtig, A.L. and Viera, C.T. (1986). Toward future research and treatment. In A.L. Hurtig and C.T. Viera (Eds), *Sickle cell disease: Psychological and psychosocial issues*. Urbana, IL: University of Illinois Press.

Hurtig, A.L. and White, L.S. (1986a). Psychosocial adjustment in children and adolescents with sickle cell disease. *Journal of Pediatric Psychology*, **11** (3), 411–427.

Hurtig, A.L. and White, L.S. (1986b). Children and adolescents: The unexplored terrain of emotion and development. In A.L. Hurtig and C.T. Viera (Eds), *Sickle cell disease: Psychological and psychosocial issues* (pp. 24–40). Urbana, IL. University of Illinois Press.

Hurtig, A.L., Koepke, D., and Park, K.B. (1989). Relation between severity of chronic illness and adjustment in children and adolescents with sickle cell disease. *Journal of Pediatric Psychology*, **14**, 117–132.

Ihekwaba, F.N. (1980). Priapism in sickle cell anaemia. *Journal of the Royal College of Surgeons*, **25**, 133.

Iloeje, S.O. (1991). Psychiatric morbidity among children with sickle cell disease. *Developmental Medicine and Child Neurology*, **33**, 1087–1094.

Jackson, D.E. (1972). Sickle cell disease: Meeting a need. *Nursing Clinics of North America*, **7**, 727–741.

Jackson, R. (1973). Sickle cell anaemia. *Urban Health*, **2**, 18–19.

Jegede, R.O., Ohaeri, J.U., Bamgboye, E.A., and Okunade, A.O. (1990). Psychiatric morbidity in a Nigerian general outpatient clinic. *West African Journal of Medicine*, **9**, 177–186.

Jessop, D.J., Riessman, C.K., and Stein, R.E.K. (1988). Chronic childhood illness and maternal mental health. *Journal of Developmental and Behavioural Pediatrics*, **9**, 147–156.

Johnson, S.B. (1985). The family and the child with chronic illness. In D.C. Turk and R.D. Kerns (Eds), *Health, illness, and families: A life span perspective*. New York: John Wiley and Sons.

154

Johnson, S.B., Pollak, T., Siverstein, J.H., Rosenbloom, A.L., Spiller, R., McCallum, M., and Harkavy, J. (1982). Cognitive and behavioural knowledge about insulin dependent diabetes among children and parents. *Pediatrics*, **69**, 708–713.

Johnson, F.L., Look, A.T., Gockerman, J., Ruggiero, M.R., Dalla-Pozza, L., and Billings, F.T. (1984). Bone marrow transplantation in a patient with sickle cell anaemia. *New England Journal of Medicine*, **311**, 780–783.

Jones, S., Shickle, D.A., Goldstein, A.R., and Serjeant, G.R. (1988). Acceptability of antenatal diagnosis for sickle cell disease amongst Jamaican mothers and female patients. *West African Medical Journal*, **37**, 12–15.

Kark, J.A., Posey, D.M., Schumacher, H.R., and Ruehle, M.D. (1987). Sickle-cell trait as a risk factor for sudden death in physical training. *New England Journal of Medicine*, **317**, 781–787.

Katz, E.R. (1980). Illness impact and social reintegration. In J. Kellerman (Ed), *Psychological aspects of childhood cancer*. Springfield, IL: C.C. Thomas.

Kazak, A. (1987). Professional helpers and families with disabled children: A social network perspective. *Marriage and Family Review*, **11**, 177–191.

Kessler, R. and Cleary, R. (1980). Social class and psychological distress. *American Sociological Review*, **45**, 463–478.

King, E.H. (1981). Child-rearing practices: Child with chronic illness and well sibling. *Issues in Comprehensive Pediatric Nursing*, **5**, 105–194.

King, N.M.P. and Cross, A.W. (1989). Children as decision makers: Guidelines for pediatricians. *The Journal of Pediatrics*, **115** (1), 10–16.

Kirkpatrick, D.V., Barrios, N.J., and Humbert, J.H. (1991). Bone marrow transplantation for sickle cell anemia. *Seminars in Hematology*, **28**, 240–243.

Kodish, E., Lantos, J., Siegler, M., Kohrman, A., and Johnson, F.L. (1990). Bone marrow transplantation in sickle cell disease: The trade-off between early mortality and quality of life. *Clinical Research*, **38**, 694–700.

Konotey-Ahulu, F.I.D. (1968). Hereditary qualitative and quantitative erythrocyte defects in Ghana: An historical and geographical survey. *Ghana Medical Journal*, **7**, 118–119.

Konotey-Ahulu, F.I.D. (1991). *The sickle cell disease patient: Natural history from a clinico-epidemiological study of the first 1550 patients of Korle Bu Hospital Sickle Cell Clinic*. London: Macmillan.

Koshy, M., Entsuah, R., Koranda, A., Kraus, A.P., Johnson, R., Bellvue, R., Flournoy-Gill, Z., and Levy, P. (1989). Leg ulcers in patients with sickle cell disease. *Blood*, **74** (4), 1403–1408.

Kumar, S., Powars, D., Allen, J., and Haywood, L.J. (1976). Anxiety, self concept, and personal and social adjustments in children with sickle cell anemia. *The Journal of Pediatrics*, **88**, 859–863.

Lavigne, J.V. and Ryan, M. (1979). Psychological adjustment of siblings of children with chronic illness. *Pediatrics*, **63**, 616–627.

Leavell, S.R. and Ford, C.V. (1983). Psychopathology in patients with SCD. *Psychosomatics*, **24**, 23–27.

Lebby, R. (1846). A case of absence of the spleen. *Southern Journal of Medical Pharmacology*, **1**, 481–483.

Leikin, S.L., Gallagher, D., Kinney, T.R., Sloane, D., Klug, P., Riada, W., and the Cooperative Study of Sickle Cell Disease. (1989). Mortality in children and adolescents with sickle cell disease. *Pediatrics*, **84** (3), 500–508.

Lemanek, K.L., Moore, S.L., Gresham, F.M., Williamson, D.A., and Kelley, M.L. (1986). Psychological adjustment of children with sickle cell anemia. *Journal of Pediatric Psychology*, **11**, 397–410.

LePontois, J. (1975). Adolescents with sickle cell anaemia deal with life and death. *Social Work in Health Care*, **1**, 71–80.

LePontois, J. (1986). Adolescents with sickle cell anemia: Developmental issues. In A.L. Hurtig and C.T. Viera (Eds), *Sickle cell disease: Psychological and psychosocial issues*. Urbana, IL: University of Illinois Press.

Lester, B.F. (1986). The social support needs of parents of children with sickle cell anemia. *Dissertation Abstracts International*, **46**, 2443.

Lipowski, Z.J. (1971). Physical illness, the individual and the coping process. *Psychiatry in Medicine*, **1**, 91–98.

Lucarelli, G., Galimberti, M., Polchi, P., Angelucci, E., Baronciani, D., Giardini, C., Politi, P., Durazzi, S.M.T., Muretto, P., and Albertini, F. (1990). Bone marrow transplantation in patients with thalassemia. *New England Journal of Medicine*, **322**, 417–421.

Luzzatto, L. and Goodfellow, P. (1989). A simple disease with no cure. *Nature*, **337**, 17–18.

Markovitz, R.J. (1984). Sickle cell anemia. In H. Roback (Ed), *Helping patients and their families cope with medical problems*. San Francisco: Jossey-Bass Publications.

Marks, R.M. and Sachar, E.J. (1973). Undertreatment of medical in-patients with narcotic analgesia. *Annals of Internal Medicine*, **78**, 173–181.

Marteau, T.M. (1989). Health beliefs and attributions. In A.K. Broome (Ed), *Health Psychology: Processes and Applications*. London: Chapman and Hall.

Marteau, T.M., Bloch, S., and Baum, J.D. (1987). Family life and diabetic control. *Journal of Child Psychology and Psychiatry*, **28**, 823–834.

Martin, E. and Martin, J. (1978). *The black extended family*. Chicago: University of Chicago Press.

Maruta, T., Swanson, D.W., and Finlayson, R.E. (1979). Drug abuse and dependency in patients with chronic pain. *Mayo Clinical Practice*, **54**, 241–244.

Mason, V.R. (1922). Sickle cell anemia. *Journal of the American Medical Association*, **79**, 1318–1320.

McAdoo, H. (1978). Factors related to stability in upwardly mobile black families. *Journal of Marriage and the Family*, **40**, 761–778.

McCalman, J.A. (1990). *The forgotten people*. London: King's Fund Centre.

McGrath, P.A. (1989). *Pain in children: Nature, assessment, and treatment*. New York: the Guilford Press.

McQuay, H.J. (1989). Opioids in chronic pain. *British Journal of Anaesthesia*, **63**, 213–226.

Melzack, R. (1975). The McGill Questionnaire; major properties and scoring methods. *Pain*, **1**, 277–299.

Melzack, R. (1990). The tragedy of needless pain. *Scientific American*, **262**, 27.

Midence, K. and Shand, P. (1992). Family and social issues in Sickle Cell Disease. *Health Visitor Journal*, **65**, 441–443.

Midence, K., Fuggle, P., and Davies, S.C. (1993). Psychosocial aspects of sickle cell disease in childhood and adolescence: A review. *British Journal of Clinical Psychology*, **32**, 271–280.

Midence, K., Davies, S.C., and Fuggle, P. (1992a). Courage in the face of crisis. *Nursing Times*, **88** (22), 46–48.

Midence, K., Davies, S.C., and Fuggle, P. (1992b). Adaptation to adversity. *Nursing Times*, **88** (23), 38–39.

Miller, S.T., Stilerman, T.V., Rao, S.P., Abhyankar, S., and Brown, A.K. (1990). Newborn screening for sickle cell disease. *American Journal of Diseases in Childhood*, **144**, 1343–1345.

Minuchin, S., Baker, L., Rosman, B., Liebman, R., Milman, L., and Todd, T. (1975). A conceptual model of psychosomatic illness in children. *Archives of General Psychiatry*, **32**, 1031–1038.

Minuchin, S., Rosman, B., and Baker, L. (1978). *Psychosomatic families*. Cambridge, MA: Harvard University Press.

Modell, B. (1991). Implications of molecular biology in prenatal diagnosis. In C.A. Seymour and J.A. Summerfield (Eds), *Horizons in Medicine*, No. 3. London: Transmedica.

Modell, B., Ward, R.H.T., and Fairweather, D.V.I. (1980). The effect of introducing ante-natal diagnosis on the reproductive behaviour of families at risk for thalassaemia major. *British Medical Journal*, **280**, 1347–1350.

Mohammed, S. (1991). Improving health services for black populations. *Share*, **1**, 1–3.

Moise, J. (1986). Towards a model of competence and coping. In A.L. Hurtig and C.T. Viera (Eds), *Sickle cell disease: Psychological and psychosocial issues*. (pp. 7–23). Urbana, IL: University of Illinois Press.

Moos, R.H. (1984). *Coping with physical illness*. New York: Plenum.

Morgan, S.T. and Jackson, J. (1986). Psychological and social concomitants of sickle cell anemia in adolescents. *Journal of Pediatric Psychology*, **11**, 429–440.

Morin, C. and Waring, E.M. (1981). Depression and sickle cell anemia. *Southern Medical Journal*, **74**, 766–768.

Murayama, M. (1964). A molecular mechanism of sickled erythrocyte formation. *Nature*, **202**: 258–260.

Murray, N. and May, A. (1988). Painful crisis in SCD: Patients' perspective. *British Medical Journal*, **297**, 452–454.

Murray, R.F., Chamberlain, N., Fletcher, J., Hopkins, E., Jackson, R., King, P.A., and Powledge, T.M. (1980). Special considerations for minority participation in prenatal diagnosis. *Journal of the American Medical Association*, **243**, 1254–1256.

Nadel, C. and Portadin, G. (1977). Sickle cell crises: Psychological factors associated with onset. *New York State Journal of Medicine*, **77**, 1075–1078.

Nagel, R.N. (1991). The dilemma of marrow transplantation in sickle cell anemia. *Seminars in Hematology*, **28**, 233–234.

Nash, K.B. (1977). Family counselling in sickle cell anaemia. *Urban Health*, **6**, 44–47.

Nash, K.B. (1986). Ethnicity, race, and the health care delivery system. In A.L. Hurtig and C.T. Viera (Eds), *Sickle cell disease: Psychological and psychosocial issues*. Urbana, IL: University of Illinois Press.

Nash, K.B., Kramer, K.D., Hughes, M., Powell, A., and Shelley, B. (1993). *National Sickle Cell mutual help directory*. The Psychosocial Research Division, Duke—UNC Comprehensive Sickle Cell Centre, University of North Carolina, Chapel Hill.

National Association of Health Authorities (1988). *Action not words*. Report produced by the National Association of Health Authorities, Birmingham.

Newacheck, P.W., McManus, M.A., and Fox, H.B. (1991). Prevalence and impact of chronic illnesses among adolescents. *American Journal of Diseases in Childhood*, **145**, 1367–1373.

Nicholson, J. (1985). *Men and women: How different are they?* Oxford: Oxford University Press.

Nishiura, E., Whitten, C.F., and Jenkins, D. (1980). Screening for psychosocial problems in health settings. *Health and Social Work*, **5**, 22–28.

Nishiura, E., Whitten, C.F., and Thomas, J.F. (1982). *School absences and sickle cell anemia*. Paper presented at the American Public Health Association Annual Meeting, Montreal.

Noel, C. (1983). Complications of sickle cell disease: Leg ulcers. *Nursing Clinics of North America*, **18**, 155–159.

Nolan, T., Desmond, K., Herlich, R., and Hardy, S. (1986). Knowledge of cystic fibrosis in patients and their parents. *Pediatrics*, **77**, 229–235.

Oppenheim, C. (1990). *Poverty: The facts*. London: Child Poverty Action Group.

Orne, M.T. (1962). On the social psychology of the psychological experiment, with particular reference to demand characteristics and their implications. *American Psychologist*, **17**, 776–783.

Patterson, H. (1980). *Sickle cell anaemia and the monitoring of chronic illness in the school-age child*. MSc Thesis. Chelsea College, University of London.

Pauling, L., Itano, H., Singer, S. J., and Wells, I.C. (1949). Sickle cell anaemia: A molecular disease. *Science*, **110**, 543–548.

Payne, R. (1989). Pain management in sickle cell disease: Rationale and techniques. *Annals of the New York Acadamy of Sciences*, **565**, 189–206.

Perrin, J.M. and MacLean, W.E. (1988). Children with chronic illness: The prevention of dysfunction. *Pediatric Clinics of North America*, **35**, 1325–1337.

Phillips, J.R. (1976). How I cope with sickle cell anaemia. *Ebony Magazine*.

Phillips, D. (1987). Searching for a decent home: Ethnic minority progress in the post-war housing market. *New Community*, **14** (1&2), 105–117.

Piomelli, S. (1985). Chronic transfusions in patients with sickle cell disease. *American Journal of Pediatric Hematology-Oncology*, **7**, 51–55.

Piomelli, S. (1991). Sickle cell diseases in the 1990s: The need for active and preventive intervention. *Seminars in Hematology*, **28**, 227–232.

Platt, O.S., Thorington, B.D., Brambilla, D.J., Milner, P.F., Rose, W.F., Vichinsky, E., and Kinney, T.R. (1991). Pain in sickle cell disease: Rates and risk factors. *New England Journal of Medicine*, **325**, 11–16.

Pless, I.B. (1985). Clinical assessment: Physical and psychological functioning. *Pediatric Clinics of North America*, **31**, 33–45.

Pless, I.B. and Perrin, J.M. (1985). Issues common to a variety of illnesses. In N. Hobbs and J.M. Perrin (Eds), *Issues in the care of children with chronic illness*. San Francisco: Jossey-Bass Publisher.

Pless, I.B., Cripps, H.A., Davies, J.M.C., and Wadsworth, M.E.J. (1989). Chronic physical illness in childhood: Psychological and social effects in adolescence and adult life. *Developmental Medicine and Child Neurology*, **31**, 746–755.

Pocock, S.J. (1983). *Clinical trials: A practical approach*. Chichester: Wiley and Sons.

Portenoy, R.K. and Foley, K.M. (1986). Chronic use of opioid analgesics in non-malignant pain: Report of 38 cases. *Pain*, **25**, 171–186.

Porter, J. and Jick, H. (1980). Addiction rate in patients treated with narcotics. *New England Journal of Medicine*, **302**, 123.

Potrykus, C. (1991). Call for better services and universal screening. *Health Visitor*, **64**, 404–405.

Powars, D. (1975). Natural history of sickle cell disease – the first ten years. *Seminars in Haematology*, **12**, 3.

Powars, D. (1989). Diagnosis at birth improves survival of children with sickle cell anemia. *Pediatrics*, **83**, 830–833.

Prashar, U., Anionwu, E., and Brozovic, M. (1985). *Sickle cell anaemia: Who cares? A survey of screening and counselling facilities in England*. London: The Runnymede Trust.

Raphael, B. and Singh, B. (1984). Recognition of dependency in both patient and therapist, and its effect on prescribing patterns. *Australian Drug and Alcohol Review*, **3**, 269–272.

Rodgers, G.P., Dover, G.J., and Noguchi, C.T. (1990). Hematologic responses of patients with sickle cell disease to treatment with hydroxyurea. *New England Journal of Medicine*, **322**, 1037–1045.

Rosenstock, I.M. (1966). Why people use health services. *Millbank Memorial Fund Quarterly*, **44**, 94–127.

Rosenthal, R. (1969). *Artifact in behavioural research*. New York: Academic Press.

Rovet, J.F., Ehrlick, R.M., and Hope, M. (1987). Intellectual deficits associated with early onset of insulin-dependent diabetes mellitus in children. *Diabetes Care*, **10**, 510–515.

Royal College of Physicians of London (1989). *Prenatal diagnosis and genetic screening; community and service implications*. London: Royal College of Physicians.

Ruchnagel, D. (1974). The genetics of sickle cell anaemia and related syndromes. *Archives of Internal Medicine*, **133**, 595–604.

Sabbeth, B.F. and Leventhal, J.M. (1984). Marital adjustment to chronic childhood illness: A critique of the literature. *Pediatrics*, **73**, 762–768.

Sargent, J. (1983). The sickle child: Family complications. *Journal of Developmental and Behavioural Pediatrics*, **4** (1), 50–56.

Satariano, W.A. and Syme, S.L. (1981). Life changes and diseases in elderly populations: Coping with change. In McGaugh, J.L. and Kiesler, S.B. (Eds), *Aging: Biology and behaviour*. New York: Academic Press.

Satcher, D. (1976). The dimension of self-concept in sickle cell counselling. In *Proceedings of the First National Sickle Cell Educational Symposium* (pp. 98–101). Washington DC: US Department of Health, Education, and Welfare.

Satterwhite, B. (1978). Impact of chronic illness on child and family: An overview based on five surveys. *International Journal of Rehabilitation Research*, **1**, 7–15.

Schechter, N.L., Berrin, F.B., and Katz, S.M. (1988). The use of patient controlled analgesia in adolescents with sickle cell pain crisis. *Journal of Pain and Symptom Management*, **3**, 1–5.

Schmidt, J.D. and Flocks, R.H. (1971). Urologic aspects of sickle cell haemoglobin. *Journal of Urology*, **106**, 740–743.

163

Schwartz, G.E. (1981). A systems analysis of psychobiology and behaviour therapy: implications for behavioural medicine. In H. Leigh (Ed), *Special Issue on Behavioural Medicine of Psychotherapy and Psychosomatics,* **36**, 159–184.

Schwartz, G.E. (1982). Testing the biopsychosocial model: The ultimate challenge facing behavioural medicine? *Journal of Consulting and Clinical Psychology,* **50**, 1040–1053.

Sellers, E. Jr. (1975). Impact of sickle cell anaemia on attitudes and relationships amongst particular family members. *Dissertation Abstracts International,* **35**, 1752–A.

Selye, H. (1976). Forty years of stress research: Principal remaining problems and misconceptions. *Canadian Medical Association Journal,* 115, 53–57.

Serjeant, G.R. (1983). Sickle haemoglobin and pregnancy. *British Medical Journal,* **287**, 628–630.

Serjeant, G.R. (1992). *Sickle cell disease.* Oxford: Oxford University Press.

Shapiro, B.S. (1989). The management of pain in SCD. *Pediatric Clinics of North America,* **36** (4), 1029–1043.

Shapiro, E.K. and Wallace, D.B. (1987). Siblings and parents in one-parent families. *Journal of Children in Contemporary Society,* **19**, 91–114.

Shapiro, B.S., Dinges, D.F., Orne, E.C., Ohene-Frempong, K., and Orne, M.T. (1990). Recording of crisis pain in sickle cell disease. In D.C. Tyler and E.J. Krane (Eds), *Advances in pain research therapy,* vol. 15 (pp. 313–321). New York: Raven Press.

Shickle, D. and May, A. (1989). Knowledge and perceptions of haemoglobinopathy carrier screening among general practitioners in Cardiff. *Journal of Medical Genetics,* **26**, 109–112.

Shute, R.H. and Paton, D. (1992). Understanding chronic childhood illness: Towards an integrative approach. *The Psychologist,* **5**, 390–394.

Singhi, P.D., Goyal, L., Pershad, D., Singhi, S., and Walia, B.N.S. (1990). Psychosocial problems in families of disabled children. *British Journal of Medical Psychology*, **63**, 173–182.

Slaughter, D. and Anderson, P. (1985). *Caring for sickle cell anemia children: Impact of father's presence or absence on maternal coping, esteem and child esteem.* Paper presented at the 18th Annual Association of Black Psychologists Convention, Chicago, IL.

Smith, J.A. (1973). *Genetic counselling—a different view.* Paper presented at the Annual Meeting of Comprehensive Sickle Cell Centers Directors, Memphis, TN.

Smith, V.W. (1980). The impact of selected internal and external influences on successful coping among mothers of children with sickle cell disease. *Dissertation Abstracts International*, **42**, 1798–A.

Spaulding, B.R. and Morgan, S.B. (1986). Spina bifida children and their families: A population prone to family dysfunction. *Journal of Pediatric Psychology*, **11**, 359–374.

Stein, R.E.K. and Riessman, C.K. (1980). The development of an Impact-on-Family Scale: Preliminary findings. *Medical Care*, **18**, 465–472.

Stimmel, B. (1983). *Pain analgesia and addiction.* New York: Raven Press.

Streltzer, J. (1980). Treatment of iatrogenic drug dependence in the general hospital. *General Hospital Psychiatry*, **2**, 262–266.

Swift, A.V., Cohen, M.J., Hynd, G.W., Wisenbaker, J.M., Mckie, K.M., Makari, G., and McKie, V.C. (1989). Neuropsychologic impairment in children with sickle cell anemia. *Pediatrics*, **84**, 1077–1085.

Taub, A. (1982). Opioid analgesics in the treatment of chronic intractable pain of neo-plastic origin. In L.M. Kitahaha and D. Collins (Eds), *Narcotic analgesia in anesthesiology* (pp. 199–208). Baltimore, MD: Williams and Wilkins.

Tennant, F.S. and Uelman, G.F. (1983). Narcotic maintenance for chronic pain: Medical and legal guidelines. *Postgraduate Medicine*, **73**, 81–94.

Thomas, E.D., Buckner, C.D., Sanders, J.E., Papayannopoulou, T., Borgna-Pignatti, C., De Stefano, P., Sullivan, K.M., Clift, R.A., and Storb, R. (1982). Marrow transplantation for thalassaemia. *Lancet*, **ii**, 227–229.

Thomas, J., Koshy, M., Patterson, L., Dorn, L., and Thomas, K. (1984). Management of pain in sickle cell disease using biofeedback therapy: A preliminary study. *Biofeedback and Self-Regulation*, **9**, 413–420.

Thompson, R.J., Gil, K.M., Abrams, M.R., and Phillips, G. (1992). Stress, coping, and psychological adjustment of adults with SCD. *Journal of Consulting and Clinical Psychology*, **60**, 433–440.

Torkington, N.P.K. (1991). *Black health: A political issue*. London and Liverpool: Catholic Association for Racial Justice and Liverpool Institute for Higher Education.

Tritt, S. (1984). The psychological adaptation of siblings of children with chronic medical illnesses: A repeated measure analysis. *Dissertation Abstracts International*, **44** (9): 2912–2913.

Tuck, S.M. (1982). Sickle cell disease and pregnancy. *British Journal of Hospital Medicine*, **28**, 125–127.

Turk, D.C. and Kerns, R.D. (1985). *Health, illness, and families: A life-span perspective*. Chichester: Wiley and Sons.

Ungerer, J., Horgan, B., Chaitow, J., and Champion, G.B. (1988). Psychosocial functioning in children and young adults with juvenile arthritis. *Journal of Pediatrics*, **81**, 195–202.

Varni, J.W. and Walco, G.A. (1988). Chronic and recurrent pain associated with pediatric chronic diseases. *Issues in Comprehensive Pediatric Nursing*, **11**, 145–158.

Varni, J.W. and Wallander, J.L. (1988). Pediatric chronic disabilities: Hemophilia and spina bifida as examples. In D. Routh (Ed), *Handbook of Pediatric Psychology*. New York: Guilford Press.

Varni, J.W., Walco, G.A., and Katz, E.R. (1989). Assessment and management of chronic and recurrent pain in children with chronic diseases. *Pediatrician*, **16**, 56–63.

166

Vavasseur, J. (1977). A comprehensive program for meeting psychosocial needs of sickle cell anaemia patients. *Journal of the National Medical Association*, **69**, 335–339.

Vermylen, C., Fernandez-Robles, E., Ninane, J., and Cornu, G. (1988). Bone marrow transplantation in five children with sickle cell anaemia. *Lancet*, **i**, 1427–1428.

Vichinsky, E.P. (1991). Comprehensive care in sickle cell disease: Its impact on morbidity and mortality. *Seminars in Hematology*, **28**, 220–226.

Vichinsky, E.P., Johnson, R., and Lubin, B.H. (1982). Multidisciplinary approach to pain management in SCD. *The American Journal of Pediatric Hematology and Oncology*, **4**, 328–333.

Walco, G.A. and Dampier, C.D. (1987). Chronic pain in adolescent patients. *Journal of Pediatric Psychology*, **12** (2), 215–223.

Walco, G.A. and Dampier, C.D. (1990). Pain in children and adolescents with sickle cell disease: A descriptive study. *Journal of Pediatric Psychology*, **15** (5), 643–658.

Walco, G.A. and Varni, J.W. (1991). Chronic and recurrent pain: Hemophilia, juvenile rheumatoid arthritis, and sickle cell disease. In J.P. Bush and S.W. Harkins (Eds), *Children in pain: Clinical and research issues from a developmental perspective* (pp. 297–315). New York: Springer-Verlag.

Wang, W.C., Parker, L.J., George, S.L., Harber, J.R., Presbury, G.J., and Williams, J.A. (1985). Transcutaneous electric nerve stimulation (TENS) treatment of sickle cell painful crises. *Blood*, **66** (Suppl. 1), 67a.

Weiss, J.O. (1981). Psychosocial stress in genetic disorders: A guide for social workers. *Social Work Health Care*, **6** (4), 17–31.

Weissman, D.E. and Haddox, J.D. (1989). Opioid pseudoaddiction—an iatrogenic syndrome. *Pain*, **36**, 363–366.

Welch, G.H. and Larson, E.B. (1989). Cost-effectiveness of bone marrow transplantation in acute nonlymphocytic leukemia. *New England Journal of Medicine*, **321**, 807–812.

Wethers, D.L. (1982). Problems and complications in the adolescent with sickle cell disease. *American Journal of Pediatric Hematology and Oncology*, **4**, 47–53.

Whitten, C.F. and Fischoff, J.F. (1974). Psychosocial effects of sickle cell disease. *Archives of Internal Medicine*, **133**, 681–689.

Whitten, C. F. and Nishiura, E.N. (1985). Sickle cell anemia. In N. Hobbs and J.M. Perrin (Eds), *Issues in the care of children with chronic illness*. (pp. 236–260). San Francisco: Jossey-Bass.

Williams, I., Earles, A.N., and Pack B. (1983). Psychological considerations in sickle cell disease. *Nursing Clinics of North America*, **18**, 215–229.

World Health Organization Advisory Group on Hereditary Diseases (1985). *Community approaches to the control of hereditary diseases*. Unpublished WHO document HMG/WG/85.10 (Can be obtained free of charge from The Hereditary Diseases Programme, WHO, Geneva, Switzerland.)

Wyatt, H.V. (1988). Improving care for people with sickle cell disease. *Health Education Journal*, 47 (2/3), 70.

Zeltzer, L., Dash, J., and Holland, J.P. (1979). Hypnotically induced pain control in sickle cell anemia. *Pediatrics*, **64**, 533–536.

Index